W9-CKJ-749

SHAPE TRAINING

The 8-Week Total Body Makeover

INCREASE TONE, MUSCLE DEFINITION, AND CARDIOVASCULAR FITNESS

Robert Kennedy,
Publisher of *MuscleMag International*,
and
Maggie Greenwood-Robinson

CB
CONTEMPORARY BOOKS
A TRIBUNE COMPANY

Library of Congress Cataloging-in-Publication Data

Kennedy, Robert, 1938–
    Shape training : the 8-week total body makeover / Robert Kennedy
and Maggie Greenwood-Robinson.
       p.   cm.
   ISBN 0-8092-3251-0
   1. Reducing exercises. 2. Exercise for women. 3. Physical
fitness for women. I. Greenwood-Robinson, Maggie. II. Title.
RA781.6.K46 1996
613.7´1—dc20   96-12824
                                                CIP

Cover design by Todd Petersen
Cover photo and interior exercise photos by Jim Amentler
Illustrations by Robert Bruce
Interior design by Hespenheide Design

Copyright © 1996 by Robert Kennedy and Maggie Greenwood-Robinson
All rights reserved
Published by Contemporary Books, Inc.
Two Prudential Plaza, Chicago, Illinois 60601-6790
Manufactured in the United States of America
International Standard Book Number: 0-8092-3251-0
10   9   8   7   6   5   4   3   2   1

Contents

Acknowledgments

Our heartfelt thanks and appreciation go to the many people who have helped make this book possible:

- Rick Balkin, our literary agent
- Kara Leverte and the staff at Contemporary Books, our publisher
- Jim Amentler, who shot the exercise and cover photographs for this book
- Gold's Gym of Venice, California, and Chicago, Illinois, where the exercise photographs were shot
- The exercise models for this book: Michelle Bellini, Monica Brandt, Marla Duncan, Amy Fadhli, Jennifer Goodwin, Monica Guerra, Debbie Kruck, Heidi Neubauer, Kimiko Tanaka, and Amy Zych
- John Parrillo, Susan M. Kleiner, Ph.D., and Cliff Sheats, the nutrition experts we have had the pleasure of working with over the years
- Ben and Joe Weider, for their combined efforts and contributions in all areas of fitness

How to Use Shape Training

How much of your figure can you reasonably change? A lot more than you think! You just need the right program. You need "shape training."

Shape Training is a workout program tailored to your *body type*—your bone structure, percentage of fat to muscle, and overall proportions. In this book, we describe the body in terms of six different types: the A-frame, H-frame, I-frame, O-frame, T-frame, and X-frame. We've crafted an exercise routine to go with each type.

The advantage of shape training compared to other exercise programs is that it treats your body as a total package and reshapes it accordingly. For example, let's say your thighs and buttocks need slimming down. You do specific exercises for those trouble spots, along with aerobics to burn fat. To offset your larger lower body, you also include building-up exercises for your shoulders, giving your body more shapely contours. Shape training transforms your figure in ways you never thought possible, leaving you with better proportions, less body fat, greater muscle tone and development, and more.

If you're consistent, you'll get results. Based on our experience with people who use these techniques, here's what you can reasonably expect from shape training month by month:

After One Month

- Fat loss of up to 10 pounds
- Loss of inches
- Lean muscle gain of a few pounds
- Better muscle definition
- Strength gains of up to 20%

After Two Months

- Positive changes in body shape
- Additional fat loss
- Additional gain in lean muscle
- Increased energy and endurance
- Greater strength
- Overall sense of well-being

After Three Months

- Further fat loss
- Lean muscle gain of up to 5 pounds (or more, depending on your metabolism)
- Increased strength (by as much as 60% compared to the start of the program)
- Improved aerobic fitness and cardiovascular efficiency
- Faster metabolism
- Reversal of some of the physical signs of aging
- Positive feelings about yourself and your body

Initially, you should follow the shape-training routine that matches your body type. After a month or two, you can switch to other workouts as your body shape changes. If you have a lot of body fat to lose, for example, you'll derive benefits from the fat-burning routines featured in the O-frame chapter. Or if you need to slim and shape your thighs, then the A-frame chapter has some good advice for you. If trimming the waistline is your goal, you'll learn how in the H-frame chapter. Or you may want to build more curves into your figure. The routine for I-frames shows you how.

Once you've changed and fine-tuned your shape, you can try the X-frame routine, an excellent, all-purpose workout designed for figure maintenance. In Appendix A, there's even a discussion of shape training during pregnancy. Also, please pay particular attention to Chapter 13, which covers nutrition for losing body fat and developing lean, shapely muscle. In short, you can learn something from every chapter in this book, regardless of your body type.

The women photographed for this book represent the "new look" in fitness. They are not overdeveloped bodybuilders, but active women who exercise for shape, tone, definition, and cardiovascular fitness. This highly sought-after look is achieved by training for shape—putting the right mix of weight training, special exercise principles, and aerobics into a workout that's targeted for your body type. As many women are, we hope you'll be motivated by these photographs. Use them to help visualize how you want your own body to look.

So there you have it. As long as you stick to the shape-training principles provided here, you'll be pleased with the results. A new body is on the way!

The exercise and nutrition instructions in this book are in no way intended as a substitute for medical consultation with your physician. Consult your physician before starting any exercise program or diet. The authors and publisher disclaim any liability or loss in connection with the exercise and nutrition advice herein.

SHAPE
TRAINING

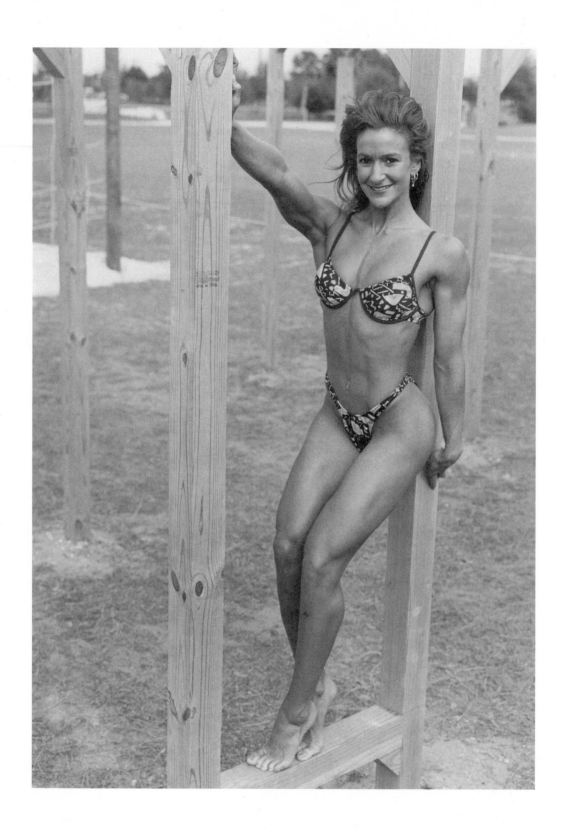

A Shortcut to Shape

Have you ever wished you could do some major remodeling on your body—like scaling down your thighs or adding to your bustline? Have you ever wanted to look more balanced, with well-shaped muscles and a proportional figure?

Good news: You can change your shape—and do it fast—with "shape training"—a unique workout that's tailored to your body type.

Like a lot of people, you've probably gone to a gym or health spa and been handed a routine to follow. That's fine, except that everybody gets the same workout. But every body is different. Therein lies the problem. You might want to trim your waistline, while your best friend is set on whittling away her hips. What works for someone else might not work for you.

Maybe that's why you're not getting results from your workout.

Maybe your workout isn't the best one for your body.

Cookie-cutter approaches to fitness don't work very well. You need a plan customized for your body. That's what shape training is all about. It works faster and better because it's tailored just for you.

Will Shape Training Help Me Spot-Reduce?

You've probably heard that spot reduction isn't possible—that when you exercise, you use energy by metabolizing fat from all over the body, not just from specific areas being worked. That's a true statement. However, blood circulation to fatty areas of the body is often sluggish. Consequently, fat is more difficult to metabolize in those spots. Exercise to the rescue! By contracting

Mia Finnegan, Ms. Fitness Olympia, exercises for shape and proportion.

muscles close to fat storage areas, you increase circulation there. The improved circulation helps pry loose stubborn fat. So there may be something to spot reduction after all. However, more research is needed.

When you look in the mirror, it's natural to hone in on body parts you don't like—say, saddlebags, a bulging tummy, or flabby upper arms. So you try to improve the areas that fall short of perfection.

The problem is, exercise programs that concentrate only on trouble spots don't work. You've got to redesign the total package. That's what shape training does—adds a bit here, takes some away there. Before long, a more balanced shape emerges. No body parts are over-developed or underdeveloped at the expense of others. Shape training reshapes your figure with an exercise program customized for your individual body type. Each routine looks at the total picture and remodels your figure in attractive ways.

How you achieve this depends largely on the way you exercise. Using a combination of weight-training exercises, aerobics, and special exercise techniques, you can shape-train certain body parts—and remodel your entire figure in the process. Simply target the muscles of those areas in your workout and challenge them accordingly. You give out-of-shape muscle groups extra attention, firm up soft spots, and

add and subtract inches where you want to.

Intensity—level of effort—is equally important. For example, to tone and tighten muscles without adding size, exercise with moderate weights for as many repetitions as you can. If you train with progressively heavier weights and lower repetitions, your muscles become fuller and more defined. You can add muscle size where you need extra curves.

Shape training not only gives you curvier muscles, it also helps you get rid of unwanted fat by developing lean muscle. Firm, strong muscles are *metabolically active*. This means they can burn calories more efficiently than body fat or untoned muscle, even at rest.

By including aerobics in your shape-training routine, you more than double your fat-burning power. In fact, a recent study found that people who combined weight-training exercises with aerobics lost two and a half times more body fat than those who performed aerobics only!

Will Shape Training Give Me the Ideal Body?

At the outset, let's scrap the notion that there's such a thing as an "ideal" shape. Sure, there are some desirables: a small waist, tiny hips, slender, toned legs, nice bustline.

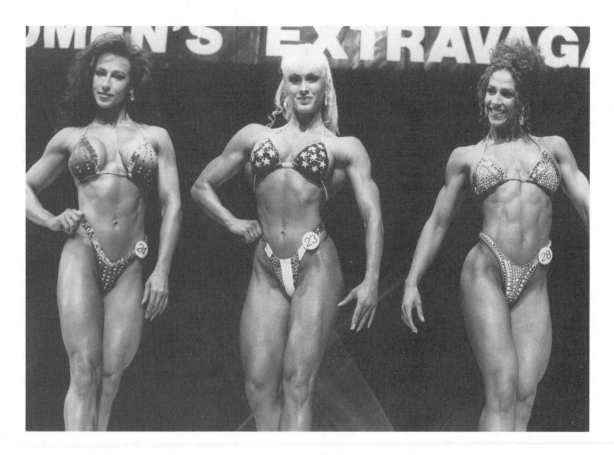

Debbie Kruck (middle) used to be a size 14 until she started training for shape.

You might also argue that any woman with those traits was just born that way. If so, you'd be right—but only partially right.

If you've ever watched some of the fitness pageant competitions on television or seen pictures of fitness models in magazines, you've seen plenty of "ideal" shapes. In fact, the women pictured in this book might look like ideals to you. Truthfully, though, each one has a very different shape. Many were even overweight at some point in their lives. Ms. Fitness USA Debbie Kruck, for example, used to be a size 14. Her hus-band called her "a fat girl with cel-lulite." Then she started a serious exercise program, trimming down to 129 firm pounds and becoming one of today's top fitness stars.

Another plump-to-perfect story is Jana Garry, a recent Ms. Hawaiian Tropic and a model for our *Muscle-Mag Video Magazine*. At 5'6" she once weighed 185 pounds. While in beauty college, she was told she had a pretty face and should become a model. But there was the problem of her weight. Determined to change, she started a regular routine of aerobics and weight training, while watching her diet. Before long, 50 pounds had melted off, and the modeling offers poured in.

Women like Debbie and Jana seem to have the ideal figure. But in reality, they've been able to recast their figures from some starting point and make some drastic changes in the way they look. And you can do the same—by training for shape.

What Can I Reasonably Change on My Figure with Shape Training?

You can't alter your inherited body frame or bone structure (although regular exercise does build bone thickness). But you can use shape training to sculpt a pleasing, aesthetic shape from what you were born with. How? In two ways: by shedding body fat and controlling lean muscle.

Let's talk about body fat first. You have about twenty to thirty billion fat cells in your body. Some of this fat is *essential fat*. It's the structural constituent of vital body parts such as the brain, nerve tissue, bone marrow, heart, and cell membranes. Women have about 12 to 15 percent essential fat.

You're probably more familiar with the other type of fat: *storage fat*. It's what we're always trying to get rid of. Some storage fat pads organs for protection. But most is found just under the skin. The distribution of storage fat on your body is called *fat patterning*. It determines your overall shape.

When you put on fat weight, storage fat cells become stuffed with fat and enlarge as a result. If you gain 50 pounds or more, fat cells start to multiply, and you've got them for life. Dieting doesn't obliterate fat cells either. It only shrinks them.

Fat cells fight to keep their size, even when you go on a diet. This may have something to do with your *setpoint,* an internal regulator that keeps your weight constant. Some scientists believe that fat cells are responsible for maintaining the setpoint by diverting energy in the form of calories away from the muscles and into fat tissues. What's more, this response may make you feel hungrier. Because so much energy is going to fat storage, your body needs extra fuel for muscles and organs. Your hunger signal turns on, and you eat more.

Women's fat cells are unlike men's in that they're controlled by different hormones and enzymes. You have more fat cells in your hips and thighs, while men have more in their abdomen. But after

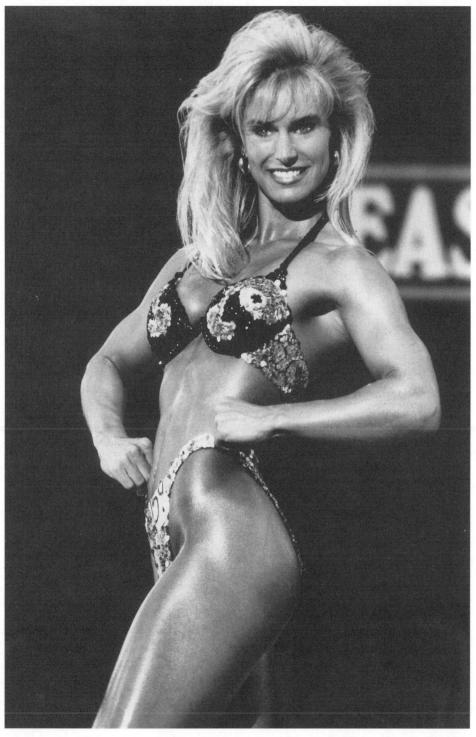

Shape training boosts your metabolism so you can stay lean and shapely.

menopause, as levels of certain hormones drop off, more fat is deposited around your midsection.

How Does Shape Training Fight Fat?

Shape training fights fat in two major ways: by burning calories and increasing your metabolism. First, shape training uses up energy in the form of calories. It offsets your "energy equation" so that energy output (exercise) is greater than energy input (calories). Shape training gets your muscles moving and your heart pumping—two actions that force your body to start breaking down fat for energy.

The amount of calories you burn per minute depends on your activity at the time. Weight training, for example, burns about 7 calories a minute, while moderate to intense aerobics such as aerobic dancing or running expends up to 12 calories a minute.

Over the long term, you can lose quite a bit of body fat with regular exercise. One pound of body fat contains about 3,500 calories. If you jogged just two miles every day for a month, you'd burn about 6,000 calories—almost two pounds of body fat. In a year, that's 24 pounds.

Second, shape training boosts your *metabolic rate*—the speed at which your body breaks down stored fat and carbohydrate for energy. Metabolic rate differs from person to person. At times, that seems unfair. Your thin-as-a-rail best friend can eat anything she wants and not gain an ounce. By contrast, you take a bite of pie, and the pounds seem to pile on. Your friend's metabolism burns up those excess calories as heat, while yours stores them as fat. But don't despair. Shape training helps rev up your metabolism.

Your total metabolic rate is really made up of three interrelated factors: basal metabolic rate, resting metabolic rate, and exercise metabolic rate. Your *basal metabolic rate* (BMR) represents the energy your body needs just to exist—to control vital internal functions such as breathing, heartbeat, the secretion of hormones, and the activity of the nervous system. The older you get, the lower your BMR gets. This drop-off is partially due to loss of muscle tissue as you age or become more inactive. Also, a woman's BMR is about 10 to 15 percent lower than a man's, simply because men have more muscle and less body fat.

But here's the real news: By increasing your ratio of lean mass to body fat, shape training helps elevate your BMR. Regardless of sex, the more muscle you have, the higher your BMR. As noted earlier, muscle is the body's most metabolically active tissue. For every new pound of muscle you put on with exercise, you use about 50 to 100 more calories a day.

You can eat more and not gain weight because you burn more, even while sleeping. Poor muscular development, on the other hand, makes it easy for your body to store fat.

Your *resting metabolic rate* (RMR) includes the BMR plus energy needed for nonexercise activities like digestion, stress responses, reactions to heat and cold, and sitting. Interestingly, one key factor in increasing the RMR is your diet. After you have eaten a meal, your RMR goes up by about 8 to 10 percent, mostly because digestion is a calorie-burning activity. That's why many nutritionists recommend eating several small meals throughout the day—to keep the RMR elevated. The type of food you eat also affects your RMR. Protein, for example, produces the greatest rise in your RMR, compared to carbohydrates or fat.

Your *exercise metabolic rate* (EMR) represents the increase in total metabolism during exercise. If you're not very active, your EMR accounts for just 12 percent of your daily energy expenditure. But if you're active, your EMR may account for 30 percent or more of your daily energy output. So the more you exercise, the more you stimulate your metabolism—in addition to the hundreds of calories you're burning during the activity. Also, depending on how hard and how long you work out, exercise can keep your RMR elevated for as long as 24 hours after exercise.

How Does Shape Training Help Control Muscle?

Along with body fat, lean muscle is the second controllable component of your shape. In fact, you can make the most significant changes in your shape in your muscles. You accomplish this by using weights to sculpt and firm your body.

Exercising with weights adds extra shape. Muscles gain new height and tone from specific exercises. Reshaping comes from concentrating on certain areas, while allowing other areas to shrink by doing less work.

Some other interesting changes take place inside your muscles, too. High-repetition weight training (15 or more reps) actually increases the ability of certain types of muscle fibers to burn more fat. Scientists have seen proof of this under the microscope by comparing women's muscle tissue before and after a period of high-repetition weight training. How do you take advantage of this knowledge? By incorporating high repetitions in your shape-training workouts, as we explain in several of the routines.

Once you start shape training, your body composition shifts to firmness and away from fat. Muscles that have been toned through shape training seem to hold any residual body fat in place better so that it "jiggles" less. Toned muscles also iron out those dimply pockets of fat known as cellulite, thus improving overall skin tone.

At first, you might be a little reluctant to exercise with weights. Many women are afraid of building bulky muscles. That's a fear we must dispel. With a consistent program of shape training, you'll develop muscle tone, not muscle bulk.

How do you know which exercises to use and how to train? By selecting the appropriate shape-training routine for your body type, then following that routine consistently. You'll learn how to identify your particular body type in the next chapter.

How Can I Get Started?

If you haven't exercised in a long time, you'll need to take a few precautions before starting the shape-training program. To begin with, be sure you have no preexisting medical problems that could be aggravated by exercise. Always check with your physician before beginning any exercise program. This is important, particularly in programs involving aerobic exercise. Aerobic workouts stress the cardiovascular system, namely the heart and blood vessels.

Also, start at a lower level of intensity. If your shape-training routine recommends jogging, for example, you should walk instead. If the routine suggests performing

four exercise sets, cut down to two or three. Progress gradually on your program. We explain how to do this in the description of each shape-training routine.

If you're new to weight training, we suggest that you work with a qualified personal trainer who can show you the ropes while you follow the instructions in this book.

Must I Diet While Following the Shape-Training Program?

Dieting as we know it is really on its way out. Most "diets" are unbalanced and calorie-restrictive. They do more harm than good, actually leading to poor health and disease. The wisest course of action is to follow a prudent diet that emphasizes food choice over food restriction. Food choice has more to do with weight control than any other factor. By selecting wholesome, close-to-nature foods, you can make a huge difference in the way you look and feel—without making major cutbacks in calories.

Here's what we mean: Nutritionists used to think that a calorie was a calorie was a calorie. But now they know better. Calories from fat head straight to the tummy and hips. It really is better to eat oatmeal or a sweet potato than ice cream or pizza! That's because fat from food is chemically similar to fat in the body and thus easy to store. Many studies have shown that overweight people prefer foods higher in fat and sugar. An excess of these foods can make the pounds pile on.

Let's say you eat 100 extra calories from a fatty food like candy or french fries. Your body may burn just 3 of those fat calories and stockpile the rest as body fat. In other words, 97 percent of all fat calories are turned into body fat.

But if you eat 100 additional calories from a complex carbohydrate such as rice or sweet potatoes, you burn 23 of those calories. The rest is put away in the liver or muscles as glycogen (the body's storage form of carbohydrate), awaiting use as energy for activity or exercise. The point is, your body handles fat calories differently than it does carbohydrate or protein calories.

By limiting the amount of fat and eating "good" calories, you can whittle away body fat without cutting calories. In Chapter 13, we outline some easy-to-follow dietary principles to help you get in shape—and stay there.

Reshaping the body is in large part a result of losing body fat and firming up muscle. When you diet and exercise properly, you let your natural shape show through.

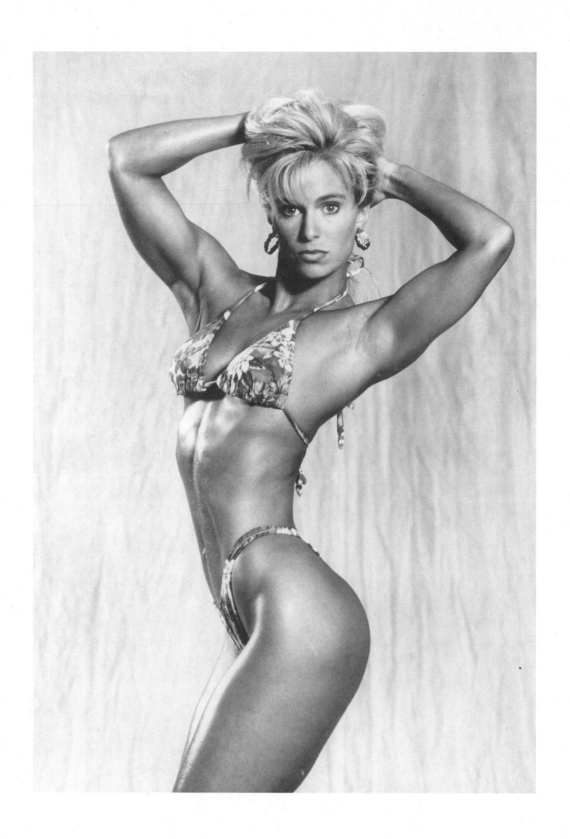

2

Size Up Your Size

Do you step on the scales to size up your figure? Most people do, even though scales aren't the best indicator of fitness. Or maybe you've used height/weight charts to compare your weight with that of other women of your height.

One of the better-known charts is the Metropolitan Life Insurance Company tables of desirable weights. Revised in 1983 to allow everyone an extra seven to ten pounds, the MetLife tables give desirable ranges of body weight for three body frames—small, medium, and large. However, many medical experts and major health associations argue that such tables are too lenient. They're based on the death rates and vital statistics of insurance policy holders, a selective group that may not reflect the average population.

A scale can be misleading as well. It tells you just one thing: your

weight. For a muscular person, 150 pounds might be perfect. For someone else, this might be dangerously overweight. Plus, if you gain a pound or more, that gain might be lean mass—exactly what you want for a great shape. Neither scales nor height/weight charts give the best picture of whether you're tubby or toned.

How Much Body Fat Should I Have?

As mentioned in the previous chapter, you need a certain amount of essential fat for good health—about 12 to 15 percent of your total weight. But too much storage fat can compromise your appearance and your health, as can too little. Here are some guidelines to give you an idea of how much fat is desirable on women:

Brandi Carrier has the right stuff: lean muscle and low body fat.

Rating (for Women)	Amount of Body Fat
Excellent	10%–15%
Good	16%–19%
Acceptable	20%–24%
Too fat	25%–29%
Obese	30% or over

How Do I Know How Much Body Fat I Have?

In addition to scales and height/weight charts, other techniques can help you take stock of your shape. Some of the most accurate methods are body composition analysis, the pinch test, and waist/hip ratios.

Body composition analysis tells you the composition of your weight, particularly how much is lean muscle and how much is pure fat. Health clubs, gyms, and fitness centers often offer body composition analysis as part of their services. Many techniques are available to analyze your body composition, some fairly simple and others quite complex. The table on page 14 summarizes pros and cons of the methods that are now most widely used.

Skinfold Technique

The *skinfold technique* measures fat just under the skin. As many as 10 sites may be measured, although the combined measurement of the abdomen, triceps, chest, and thigh skinfolds is usually enough for an accurate reading. Skinfolds are mea- sured by a set of calipers, a device that pinches up folds of fat away from the underlying muscle tissue. The measurements are plugged into a formula that calculates percentages of body fat and lean mass.

When it comes to accuracy, this rather low-tech technique stacks up well against higher-tech measurement tools. In a study at the University of British Columbia, researchers compared the skinfold technique to two other methods of body composition testing: ultrasound and computed tomography, better known as a CT scan. (CT scanners combine x-rays with computer technology to provide clear, cross-sectional images of fat and nonfat tissue. Because of their accuracy and reliability, CT scans are considered by many to be the gold standard for body composition testing. Realistically, though, they are impractical because of their high cost and inconvenience, so their present use is limited to research settings.) In the study, 13 men and 9 women had their body composition analyzed at three abdominal sites by skinfold calipers, CT scans, and ultrasound. Amazingly, the skinfold measurements matched the CT measurements more closely than the ultrasound measurements did.

The accuracy of the skinfold technique depends on the skill of the person performing the measurements and the number of sites measured. For best results, it's advisable

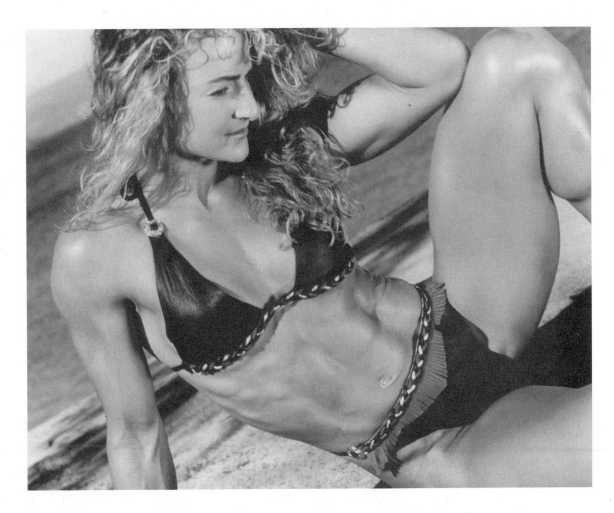

to have your skinfolds measured by a skilled technician. Use the same person each time, too. The skinfold technique does not work well with very obese people. Most calipers are not large enough to measure their skinfold thicknesses.

Ultrasound

With *ultrasound*, a popular body composition technique, equipment sends ultrasound waves through the skin and measures underlying fat and muscle. Typically, scans of body fat are taken in several areas of the body. Measurements of body fat thickness can then be taken to calculate total fat.

Experts disagree about the accuracy of ultrasound. Some rate it as accurate; others say it's less precise than other methods of body composition testing.

Bioelectrical Impedance Analysis

To use *bioelectrical impedance analysis* (BIA), the technician passes a painless electrical current through

Mia Finnegan is lovely—and lean.

Techniques for Body Composition Testing

Technique	Length of Test	Accuracy	Convenience	Cost
Skinfold technique	10 or more minutes, depending on how many sites are measured	High (though not indicated for very obese people). Different results may be obtained by different examiners.	Very convenient. Can be done at home.	Inexpensive. A set of calipers costs approximately $20; however, prices vary.
Ultrasound	10 minutes, on average	Moderate	Fairly convenient. Performed at health clubs, doctors' offices, or clinics.	$20, on average
Bioelectrical impedance analysis (BIA)	Depending on the instrument, from as little as a few seconds to much longer	Moderate to high. Does not do a good job of measuring body fat in the trunk of the body.	Fairly convenient. Performed at health clubs, doctors' offices, or clinics.	Low ($25–$50); however, BIA-type scales cost $500.
Underwater weighing	Time-consuming	High	Highly inconvenient; requires a great deal of cooperation. Performed at universities and sports-medicine complexes.	High
Infrared interactance	From a few seconds to much longer, depending on how many sites are measured	Moderate	Fairly convenient. Performed at health clubs, doctors' offices, or clinics.	Low
BOD POD Body Composition System	Very brief	More scientific data needed to confirm accuracy	Convenient, if your health club has the technology	$25–$100

the body. The current is introduced at electrodes placed on the hands and feet. Fat tissue won't conduct the current, but fat-free tissue (namely water) will. The faster the current passes through the body, the less body fat there is. Readings obtained from the test are put into special formulas adjusted for height, sex, and age to calculate percentages of body fat and fat-free mass.

Some newer BIA devices resemble bathroom scales with electrodes on the pad. You simply step on the pad, and the device measures your body composition instantly. It then displays and prints out your weight, body fat, total body water, and muscle.

One drawback of BIA is that most of the electrical conduction occurs in the limbs. It therefore may be less helpful for measuring body fat in the trunk.

Underwater Weighing

Usually reserved for research studies, *underwater weighing* positions you in a chair suspended from a scale. After exhaling, you're dunked in a tank of water and required to hold your breath for about 10 seconds while your weight under water is measured. The entire procedure is repeated several times. The three heaviest readings are averaged and put into a set of equations to figure out your percentage of body fat.

Obviously, this is a lot of bother. This method is also less accurate for women, due to wide variations in the amount of women's fat-free mass (bones, muscle, and other nonfat tissue).

Infrared Interactance

The *infrared interactance* technique is based on light absorption and reflection principles. A light-emitting wand is placed on various sites of the body. The energy reflected back is analyzed to estimate your body composition. In less than 10 seconds, your percentage of body fat is calculated.

Infrared interactance is safe, noninvasive, and easy to use. But despite its convenience and high-tech appeal, it has some flaws in accuracy. In one study, skinfold thicknesses measured at seven sites on the body proved to be more precise in assessing body fat than did infrared interactance. In other studies, infrared interactance overestimated body fat in lean people and underestimated body fat in obese people.

BOD POD System

The *BOD POD Body Composition System* uses computerized sensors to figure out how much air is displaced while you're sitting in a special compartment. A calculation is then made to determine your percentage of body fat. To date, only a few health clubs have this technology.

What If I Don't Have Access to Body Composition Techniques?

Even if you don't have access to these techniques, you can track your own body composition. A great way to do this is to use a simple tape measure and take *body circumference measurements*. At the same place each time, measure the circumference of (distance around) your upper arm, chest, waist, hips, and thighs. Record these numbers and watch them change for the better as you shape-train.

A variation of using these measurements is to find your *waist/hip ratio* (WHR), a measure often used by clinicians. If you gain body fat, your WHR tends to increase. Lose fat, and your WHR goes down. Here's how to calculate your WHR:

1. Measure your waist at your belly button.
2. Measure your hips at their widest point. Stand with your feet apart and your abdomen relaxed.
3. Divide your waist measurement by your hip measurement. The result is your WHR.

Ideally, this number should be no greater than .80. If it is, you need to trim down.

Another easy-to-do method is the *pinch test*. This tells you very quickly whether you've got too much extra padding. Here's how to do this test:

1. Pinch a fold of skin and fat at the back of your upper arm over the triceps muscle area. Don't pinch the triceps muscle itself.
2. Remove your fingers, but maintain the "measurement."

3. Measure the space between your fingers with a ruler.

If the space between your fingers measures more than an inch, then you may have some fat to shed.

If you don't want to measure or pinch, simply look in the mirror. That's right—stand nude in front of a full-length mirror and make an honest assessment of your present shape. What's it like? A thin, long-limbed frame that could use some flattering curves? A soft, round body with more body fat than you'd like? Or a figure that's naturally muscular and athletic-looking?

These are descriptions of three basic body types: the ectomorph, endomorph, and mesomorph. In the forties, a man named Dr. William H. Sheldon created this well-known and medically approved system of classifying people by body types. By photographing and measuring 46,000 men and women, Sheldon and his colleagues eventually developed 88 distinct categories. To simplify his system, he then created the three major divisions of ectomorph, endomorph, and mesomorph. Within each of these major divisions are "degrees of dominance." In other words, no one is purely ecto-morph, mesomorph, or endomorph but rather a combination of all three body types. One type, however, usually dominates the body.

Ectomorphy refers to thinness. If your body is ectomorphic, you

What's Your Body Type?

Body Type		Features
A-Frame		Medium to large bone structure; wide hips relative to shoulder width; full thighs; tendency to have lower body fat patterning; slow to moderate metabolism
H-Frame		Medium to large bone structure; broad shoulders; thick waist; full thighs and hips; nearly equal proportion of lean muscle to body fat; possible tendency to gain weight in abdominal and hip areas; moderate metabolism
I-Frame		Small bone structure; lean limbs and trunk; little muscularity; low body fat; fast metabolism
O-Frame		Large bone structure; wide hips; broad shoulders; full thighs, hips, and breasts; high percentage of body fat to lean muscle; slow metabolism
T-Frame		Small to medium bone structure; shoulder width even with hips; wide shoulders; full breasts; tendency to gain body fat in the trunk; moderate metabolism
X-Frame		Small to medium bone structure; shoulder width even with hips; small waist; full breasts; tendency to gain body fat in the hips and thighs; moderate metabolism

tend to be almost reed-slim, with small bones, long limbs, and little muscle or body fat. What's more, you probably have a fast metabolism and rarely put on body fat.

Endomorphy characterizes the amount of body fat you have. Endomorphic physiques are typically fuller and soft, with a higher ratio of body fat to muscle. Unlike

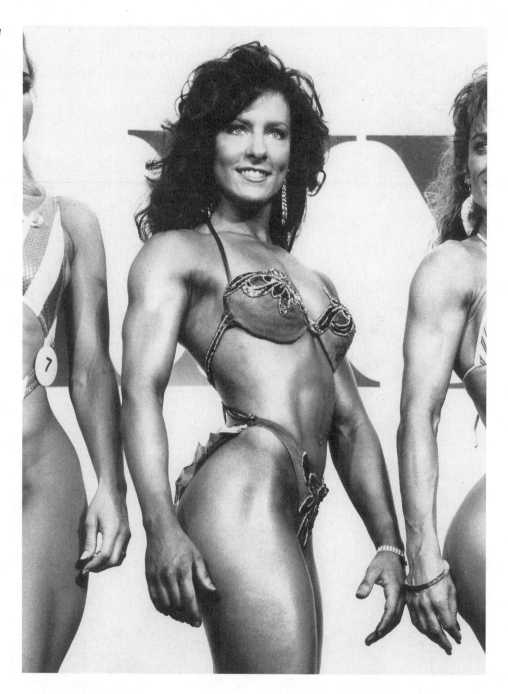

ectomorphs, endomorphs gain weight easily. Body fat is usually distributed in the hips, thighs, and buttocks.

Mesomorphy describes the degree of muscularity you have. A square body, large bones, and prominent muscular development are all features of the mesomorphic physique.

These classifications only describe tendencies toward certain characteristics. Most of us are mixtures of all three body types.

How Do I Know What My Body Type Is?

For purposes of this book, we've expanded Dr. Sheldon's three body types into six categories that better define women's bodies: the A-frame, H-frame, I-frame, O-frame, T-frame, and X-frame.

As you assess yourself in the mirror, note how your body weight is distributed. Then check the body frame descriptions given in the table titled "What's Your Body Type?"

Knowing your waist/hip ratio can help, too. Choose the frame that best approximates your present shape, then follow the shape-training program that matches your body type.

How Often Should I Analyze My Shape and Body Composition?

Whatever method you use to assess your shape, we recommend that you do some type of assessment at least twice: once when you begin the program and again after you feel you've reached your shape-training goals. Your first assessment provides the benchmark against which you'll measure your progress toward a firmer, shapelier you.

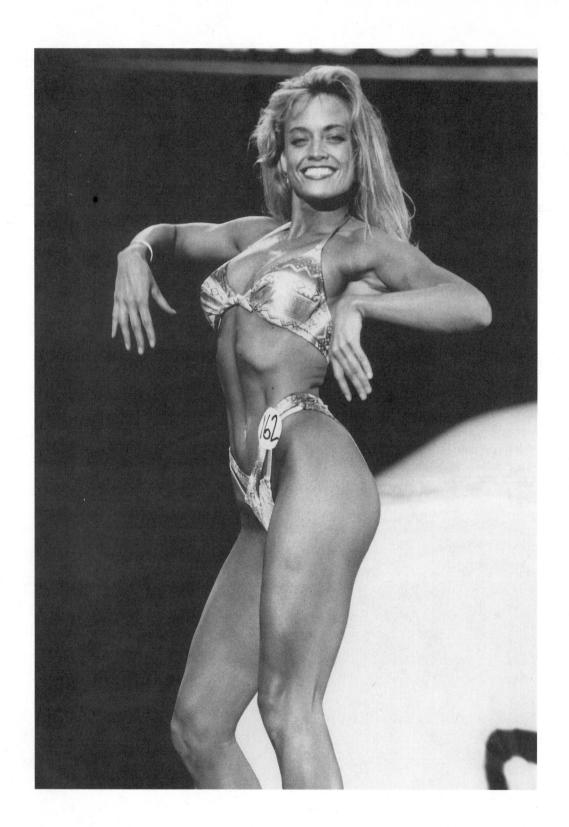

Your Health and the Shape of Fat

Where you're plump—technically known as "fat patterning"—influences more than just your appearance. It directly affects your health. People with a type of fat patterning known as *upper-body obesity* or *central obesity* are high-risk candidates for diabetes, heart disease, and certain cancers. H-frames, T-frames, and O-frames, in particular, are at risk, since they have extra pounds deposited around their upper bodies (namely the waist, chest, neck, and arms).

A-frames and some H-frames, on the other hand, tend to store fat on their hips and thighs. This type of fat patterning is called *lower-body obesity*. Though less health-risky than upper-body obesity, lower-body fat is hard to budge, setting the stage for other fat-triggered health problems.

Why Do Some People Have Paunches and Others, Saddlebags?

No one knows for sure why fat patterning differs from one person to another, but there are some theories. One has to do with hormones. Upper-body obesity is typically, but not always, a male trait. Compared to women with lower-body fat, upper-body-obese women have more male hormones, although not in large amounts. The distribution of their weight—mostly around the midsection—resembles that of paunchy men. Women with excess abdominal and upper-body fat also have higher-than-normal levels of the hormone estrogen, a risk factor for certain hormone-dependent cancers.

Scientists have discovered that the size of fat cells plays a role, too.

Staying in shape helps you stay in radiant health. (Model: Liz Worthen)

Fat cell size is regulated by *receptors* called alpha$_2$ and beta$_1$. Receptors are structures on the surfaces of cells that attach to hormones and are stimulated in the process. When the beta$_1$ receptor is stimulated, the activity of a fat-burning enzyme inside the fat cell increases. But when the alpha$_2$ receptor is stimulated, fat-burning activity is inhibited. Fat stays inside the cell, further inflating the fat cell.

In one study, scientists found that men and women both have higher alpha$_2$ activity in the buttocks than in the abdominal area—a possible reason why fat on the buttocks is so hard to shed. Men have more alpha$_2$ activity in the abdomen than women do, which could explain why men are more prone to potbellies. What the future holds for research like this is uncertain. But just think: If scientists were able to control the activity of fat cell receptors, we'd have a potentially powerful tool for spot slimming!

Another theory of body shape is that fat patterns are inherited. In other words, you're born with a genetically determined contour of padding.

Diet history plays a role, too. Women who repeatedly go on and off diets tend to have higher waist/hip ratios than those who keep their weight fairly stable. Also, high-fat diets have been shown to increase abdominal fat. So do repeated pregnancies.

But don't despair. Though all these factors are involved to some extent, you can still alter your figure by training and dieting for shape.

What's the Harm of Upper-Body Obesity?

Upper-body fat is a risk factor for a host of health problems, including problems with metabolism of blood sugar, cancers of the endometrium and breast, heart disease, and increased mortality.

Problems with Blood Sugar Metabolism

In upper-body obesity, a lot of fat is deposited around the waist. Fat cells there tend to be larger than those in other parts of the body. Large fat cells can't properly utilize blood sugar, better known as glucose. This in turn causes glucose levels to rise. In response, the pancreas secretes more of the hormone insulin. With a glut of insulin in the blood, full-blown diabetes can erupt. In fact, studies have shown that women with upper-body fat have high blood levels of insulin, sugar, and fats—all factors that can influence the development of diabetes. Plus, too much insulin may cause the kidneys to reabsorb sodium, and this can promote high blood pressure.

Endometrial Cancer

Plump women whose body fat is distributed around and above the waist run a high risk of developing endometrial cancer, one of the most common cancers that afflict women. It usually occurs after menopause, and if detected early, it's almost always curable. Scientists speculate that one reason for the risk is that upper-body-obese women have higher levels of the female hormone estrogen, which can set the stage for endometrial cancer.

In a study at the H. Lee Moffitt Cancer Center in Tampa, Florida, researchers looked into the possible link between upper-body fat and endometrial cancer. They took body fat measurements from 40 women newly diagnosed with endometrial cancer and from 40 cancer-free women. They also measured body weight and height, skinfold thicknesses, and waist/hip ratios.

The findings: A link did exist between upper-body fat and endometrial cancer. Compared to controls, the cancer patients had higher percentages of body fat, as well as higher waist/hip ratios. The researchers pointed out in their report that slimming down would be one step toward reducing the risk of endometrial cancer.

In a similar study at the National Cancer Institute, researchers examined 403 women with endometrial cancer and 297 controls to see whether body size and body fat distribution were associated with the risk of this cancer. The researchers found that women whose weight exceeded 171 pounds had 2.3 times the risk of those weighing less than 127 pounds. In addition, women with higher-than-normal waist/hip ratios had a substantial risk of developing endometrial cancer.

These and other studies point to one conclusion: The bigger the waist compared with hips and thighs, plus the higher the body fat percentage, the greater the risk of developing endometrial cancer.

Breast Cancer

Like endometrial cancer, most breast cancers have a hormonal link. In fact, estrogen can accelerate the cancer's growth. Women with

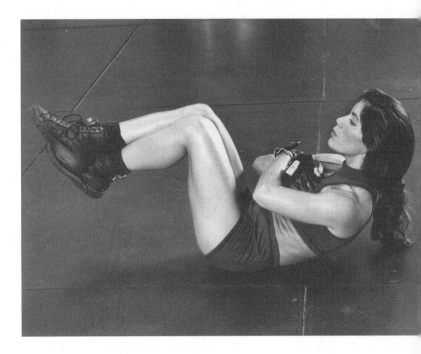

Exercising the abdominals is one way to fight a spare tire. (Model: Monica Guerra)

upper-body fat have higher levels of estrogen, and some investigators think that these women run a significantly higher risk of developing breast cancer.

That risk could go up when there's a family history of breast cancer. Researchers at the H. Lee Moffitt Cancer Center studied 56 relatives of breast cancer patients and 56 controls to detect any correlations between family history and body fat distribution. Skinfold thicknesses were taken, and waist/hip ratios were measured in all subjects. The relatives of breast cancer patients had significantly higher waist/hip ratios than the controls. This finding led the researchers to conclude that a family history of breast cancer, combined with upper-body fat, presents a significant risk for the disease.

But some investigators aren't so sure. At the Memorial Sloan-Kettering Cancer Center in New York City, 300 women had their waist and hip circumferences measured before undergoing diagnostic breast surgery. Also, the researchers took detailed risk assessments of the health and family history of each participant. Based on the data, the women were divided into three groups: those with breast cancer, those with a high risk of developing the disease, and controls. The researchers wanted to learn whether body fat distribution had anything to do with the development of can-

cer. However, they could find no trend between increasing waist/hip ratios and breast cancer risk. As for any clear-cut link, more studies need to be done before we see how this all shakes out.

Heart Disease

Not to keep piling on the bad news, but upper-body obesity is also a risk for heart disease. Research has shown that upper-body obesity results in unhealthy cholesterol profiles, high triglycerides (blood fats), and high blood pressure—which can all spell heart trouble.

Mortality

Upper-body fat is linked to a reduced life expectancy, says one study. Researchers looked at health, lifestyle, and mortality information on more than 40,000 Iowa women between ages 55 and 69 over a five-year period. The participants were mailed a questionnaire that included information about their height, weight, and weight at an earlier age. They were also asked to have their waist/hip ratios measured.

The findings were particularly worrisome. Of the 1,504 women whose deaths were reported during a follow-up period, more than 80 percent had cancer or cardiovascular disease. The rate of death among women with the highest waist/hip ratios was more than twice that of women with the lowest waist/hip ratios.

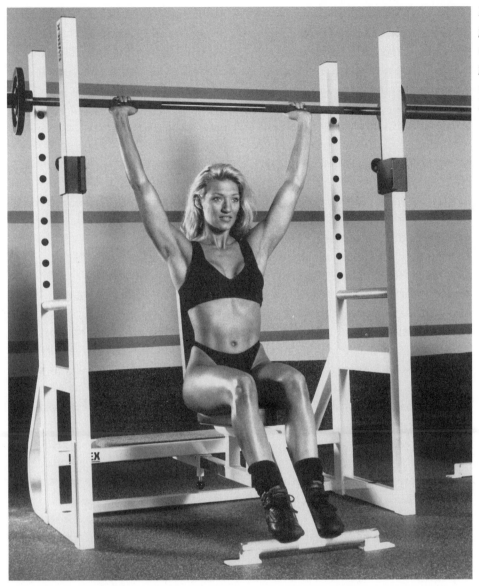

Exercise can protect against certain health problems. (Model: Heidi Neubauer)

Can Exercise Fight These Life-Shortening Illnesses?

Your body shape is not a death sentence. With vigorous exercise (and the right diet), you can shed abdominal fat more easily than body fat elsewhere. Intense exercise boosts the output of the hormone adrenaline. One of its jobs is to increase fatty acids in the bloodstream so that the body can use them for fuel. Fat cells in the abdominal area are very sensitive to adrenaline. In response to exercise, they liberate fatty acids quite readily. It's much easier to work off fat from the abs than it is from the thighs and hips, where fat cells are more stubborn.

Additionally, exercise may be protective against breast cancer. In fact, a recent TV ad campaign from an athletic shoe company reminds viewers that the risk of breast cancer is reduced when you're active from childhood on. There's a lot of truth to this, based on one large study. Investigators in California surveyed 545 newly diagnosed breast cancer patients, age 40 and younger, and 545 cancer-free controls matched for age. The survey asked the women about their exercise habits since starting menstruation.

It turns out that the women who had exercised an average of four hours a week since that time reduced their risk of breast cancer by 50 percent. Those who had exercised just one to three hours a week cut their risk by 30 percent.

The reason for this risk reduction? The scientists speculate that exercise protects breasts by altering hormone levels and decreasing ovulation—two factors known to help guard against breast cancer. The important message in here is that lifelong exercise is one possible means of preventing this dreaded disease.

As for heart disease, you can overturn some of the risk factors in as little as six weeks. That's the conclusion of a recent University of Minnesota study. Scientists placed 33 women and 8 men on a calorie-controlled, low-fat, low-salt, and high-fiber diet for six weeks with moderate exercise. On average, the participants lost 10 pounds, trimmed inches off their bodies in five places, lowered dangerous levels of cholesterol, and kept their blood pressure within normal ranges.

The lesson in all of this: Work that body hard—and consistently!

Is Lower-Body Fat as Dangerous as Upper-Body Fat?

Compared to upper-body fat, fat stored in the lower body is not as dangerous. But keep this in mind: Excess fat, regardless of where you wear it, is an unhealthy proposition.

The latest word on this comes from the Harvard Nurses' Health Study, which has followed more than 115,000 women nurses since 1976. The study suggests that being even a little on the plump side is risky to your health. Middle-aged women have the lowest risk of death if they weigh 15 percent below average, according to the study. The researchers caution, however, that this finding isn't a license to pursue an anorexic slimness. The important message in the study is that younger women should avoid weight gain early in order to prevent dangerous, hard-to-lose middle-age spread later.

Where lower-body fat is concerned, one risk is *osteoarthritis*, a disabling joint disease that affects millions of people. Any extra pounds you carry around burden your joints—a wear-and-tear effect that potentially leads to osteoarthritis. This crippling disease doesn't go away, either; it just gets worse over time.

From an appearance standpoint, the frustrating thing about lower-body fat is that it wants to stay put. This is partly nature's doing. You need that fat for menstruation, pregnancy, and lactation. It's only during lactation that the body willingly gives up lower-body fat cells, and it does this to support the energy needs of the nursing baby. In fact, research suggests that exclusively or partially breast-feeding reduces a mother's hip measurements, though this effect is only temporary.

As you move into menopause, fat starts to settle around your waist—and does so at a rather alarming rate, unless you exercise and eat right. As we already explained, this redistribution creates some life-shortening health concerns.

What Else Causes Shape to Change?

Clearly, shape changes with age. But these changes aren't due only to body fat redistribution. Unless you exercise, muscle starts withering away, too. Research suggests that low muscle weight is a risk factor for low bone mineral density. This problem can turn into *osteoporosis*, a painful thinning of the bones that can afflict women after menopause. It causes disfigurement, disability, fractures, and broken bones. Fortunately, it's preventable—particularly with muscle-strengthening exercises and a healthful, calcium-rich diet.

Changing your body for the better clearly has some dramatic, life-saving effects on your health. With shape training, some significant changes will take place on the inside, as well as on the outside.

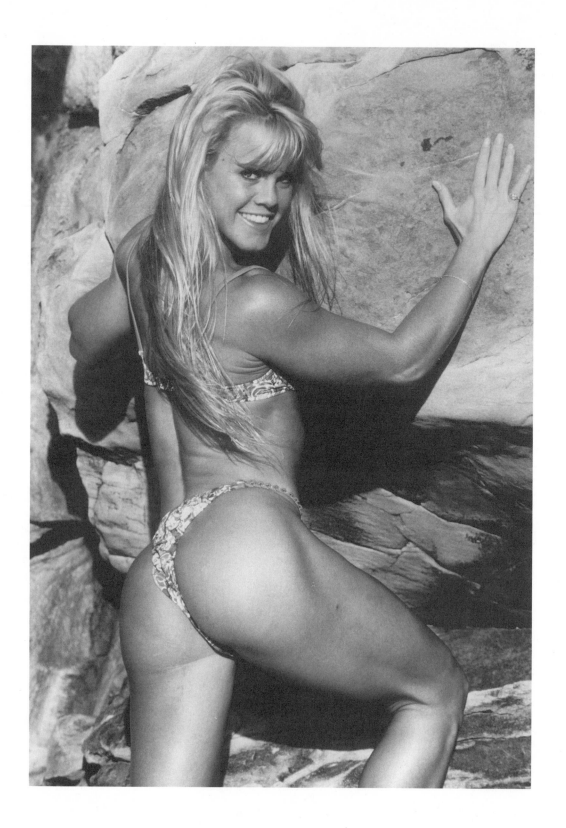

Shape-Training Basics

If you haven't gotten great results from exercise in the past, have you ever wondered why? One reason may have to do with exercise performance. How rapidly and effectively you reshape your body depends a lot upon doing your exercises correctly. What follows are some shape-training basics to help you get in shape faster.

What Kind of Equipment Should I Use?

The routines in this book employ a variety of equipment, each designed for a specific shape-training task. Barbells and dumbbells—known as *free weights*—are superior for firming up muscle and building strength in the shortest possible time. A barbell is a long, straight metal rod to which iron or vinyl sand-filled plates are attached by collars. The collars

keep the plates from sliding across the bar. Another type of barbell, called a *cambered bar,* features a wavy rod between the two plates. This design better accommodates your grip on certain arm exercises. Exercises with barbells work groups of muscles and do an excellent job of building overall strength and muscular tone. Dumbbells are simply shorter versions of barbells and are used to isolate and define specific muscles.

Most free weights are "adjustable," meaning you can switch plates according to how much weight you want to lift. Loading and unloading the plates between exercises can be time-consuming. For that reason, it's a good idea to have a few "fixed" dumbbells or barbells on hand. The plates on these weights are permanently anchored to the bar. Fixed weights are more convenient (you don't have to keep

Shannon Meteraud has toned her figure with basic shape-training techniques.

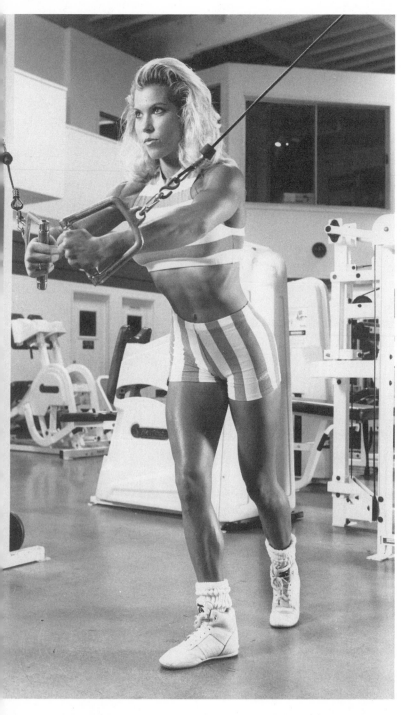

Cable equipment helps you target specific muscle groups.
(Model: Jennifer Goodwin)

changing plates), but you do need more of them. Compared to machines, free weights activate more muscles simultaneously and require greater exertion just to maintain balance and coordination.

At first, some women are intimidated by free weights and prefer to use machines instead. A word of caution: Most machines have been designed to fit a man's build and therefore don't suit a woman's body. It may feel awkward to move through the exercise and difficult to lift enough weight to make a difference. You'll have to experiment.

Machines do have some pluses, however. They allow you to work specific angles of a muscle for better body-shaping results. Also, machines provide variety.

Many of the shape-training exercises also employ cable equipment. A cable is attached by a pulley to a weight stack, which you can adjust according to the amount of weight you want to use. Cable exercises isolate specific muscles to better develop shape and definition. For versatility, you can use a variety of handles with cable exercises, including bars, ropes, and ankle straps.

Does Aerobic Equipment Play a Role in Shape Training?

Today, there's a whole new generation of high-tech aerobic equipment in gyms and health clubs, and we recommend you test-drive it. This equipment includes electronic stair-climbing machines, stationary bicycles, recumbent bicycles, and rowing machines. (These are covered in the next chapter.)

But keep in mind that the wizardry of a fancy machine is not what produces results. It's you—the human effort behind the equipment. All equipment works, if you work it hard.

How Should I Perform the Actual Shape-Training Exercise?

In shape training, the way you execute each repetition makes the difference between results that are pleasing and those that are just mediocre. By performing every rep correctly, you work your muscle fibers completely and efficiently, resulting in muscular tone, shape, and strength.

To begin with, a *repetition* is the path of an exercise from the start of the movement to the midpoint and back again to the start position. Sounds simple enough, but a lot goes into performing repetitions correctly. Here are some pointers on grip, style, speed, breathing, and concentration.

Grip
Using a narrow or wide grip on certain exercises may work certain parts of the muscle a little more, but the difference is not substantial. Choose the grip that feels most comfortable and natural to you. Your grip on the bar or the machine handle should be firm but not too tight. Squeezing the equipment wastes valuable energy that should be exerted in the exercise.

Style
Always control the exercise. A mistake many exercisers make is starting the exercise with a rapid, jerky movement. This action gives the weight so much impetus that it practically glides to the midpoint of the rep, using little muscular force to get there. As a result, the muscles encounter limited resistance. Without resistance, muscles aren't properly challenged and may not respond as well.

The correct way to start the repetition is to gradually apply the sheer force of your muscles to lift the weight. If you can't lift the weight without jerking it, then your poundage is too heavy. Try a lighter weight. Strict style and technique are more important than the amount of weight you lift.

Speed
Slow is the watchword in shape training. Both the raising motion of a lift (referred to as the *positive*) and the lowering motion (called the *negative*) should be performed slowly, in a controlled fashion. That way, you effectively isolate the muscles

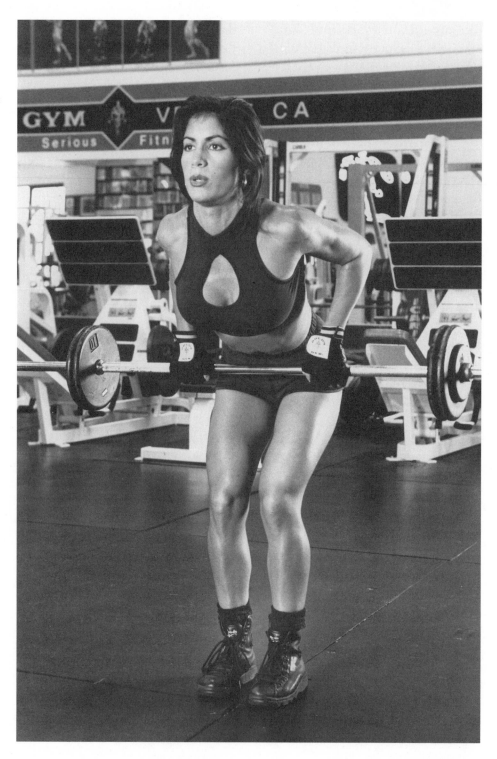

Heavier poundages add inches in the right places. (Model: Monica Guerra)

SHAPE TRAINING

being worked. Fast, jerky repetitions, on the other hand, don't isolate muscles but instead place harmful stress on the joints, ligaments, and tendons. Not only is this an unproductive way to tone muscles, it's also a dangerous training habit to adopt because it increases your risk of injury.

At the midpoint or top of the exercise, pause for a second to tense your muscles. Then lower the weight slowly again, accentuating the negative portion of the lift. This gives your muscles maximum stimulation from the exercise.

Proper Breathing

With every repetition, inhale just before the lift and exhale as you complete it. Try to synchronize inhalation and exhalation rhythmically with the motion of the rep.

Never hold your breath. Holding your breath cuts oxygen supply to the blood. Coupled with the exertion of the lift, this could cause lightheadedness or fainting.

Concentration

As you lift, concentrate on each repetition. Watch your muscles contract. Feel the sensation as they work against the resistance. Focusing on your form frees you from external distractions that could lead to sloppy, wasted repetitions.

Which Should I Increase— Resistance or Reps?

Each time you exercise, you need to challenge your muscles to work harder. Therefore, once an exercise starts feeling light, you should begin progressively upping your poundages or doing more repetitions. Muscles adapt very quickly to stresses placed on them. For continual progress, you must always add weight to the bar, do more repetitions with the same weight, or both. Increasing your effort each workout makes your muscles firmer and stronger.

Generally, to add inches to certain body parts, you'll want to increase your poundages, while keeping your repetitions in the range of 6 to 10. The poundage must be enough to stimulate the muscles, yet not so much that you start using sloppy form. Use poundages light enough to let you train in a good style, but heavy enough to tax the muscles.

Higher repetitions (12 or more) performed with moderate to heavy poundages helps put your body in a fat-burning mode. So does performing more sets. (A *set* is a series of repetitions.) Increasing the number of sets uses up more calories, thus burning fat and increasing definition and tone. Additional sets also help you develop more calorie-burning muscle.

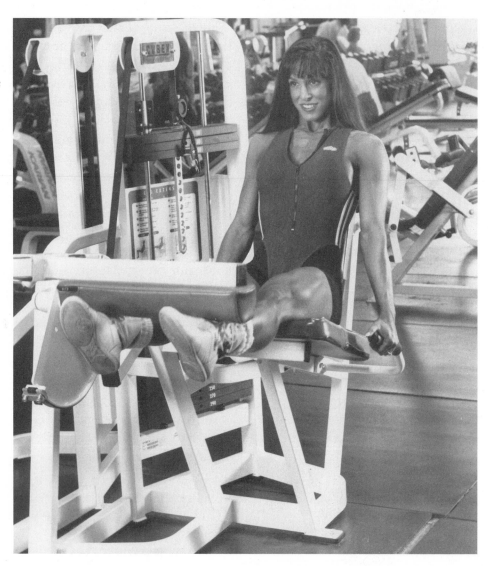

Strict exercise performance produces results. (Model: Michelle Bellini)

How Long Should I Rest Between Exercise Sets?

Generally, 30 to 60 seconds is a long enough rest between sets. However, the shorter the better. Brevity between sets produces an aerobic effect that enhances cardiovascular conditioning and stimulates fat burning. If you're trying to knock off body fat, stick to short rest periods of 30 seconds. Also, when you minimize your rest between sets, you can burn as many as 500 calories per hour.

Some leg exercises may leave you breathless after completion of a set. In that case, begin your next set after your breathing has returned to normal. If you don't wait, your cardiovascular system will outrun itself because of an accumulated oxygen debt. Resume the exercise after you've caught your breath. This may necessitate a rest period of longer than 30 seconds. Let your breathing be your guide.

In What Order Should I Do My Exercises?

There are many ways to arrange your exercises in a routine. A widely recommended method is to work large muscles groups like thighs, chest, and back first. They tax your energy reserves more than small muscles like arms do. The logic is that you're stronger and more energetic at the beginning of a workout than at the end. You'll have greater stamina for the entire workout if you start with large muscles and finish off with small ones.

In shape training, however, exercise order doesn't necessarily depend on muscle size. In some routines, you work your most underdeveloped body parts first, when your energy levels and enthusiasm are at their highest. That way, you can give your best effort to areas that need the most attention.

The shape-training routines also group together the exercises for each general area. For example, you'll follow a thigh exercise with another one for the legs. Grouping the exercises in such a fashion provides the best possible stimulation to specific body parts.

How Many Times a Week Should I Work Out?

With shape training, workout frequency depends on your body type. I-frames benefit from short, intense workouts three times a week. In contrast, if you're an O-frame or an A-frame who needs to lose body fat, we suggest that you schedule additional weekly workouts.

One way to get in additional workouts is by using a *split routine*. This means you train just one, two, or three muscle groups at a time, on certain days. Several of the shape-training workouts in this book are split routines.

Should I Use Training Aids?

There is a place in your shape-training program for training aids, such as belts, gloves, and wrist wraps. The trick is to know how and when to use them. The easiest way to explain their proper use is by discussing each one individually.

A training belt can be helpful when you're performing exercises like the squat and dead lift—two shape-training exercises that develop the body quite fast. These exercises often put the back in a compromising position, and the belt helps protect against injury.

Gloves provide a better grip on exercise bars and handles. They also help prevent your palms from developing calluses.

You don't really need to wear wrist wraps unless you're doing extremely heavy lifts—like 400-pound bench presses! Those are reserved only for power lifters. Most women can't and shouldn't attempt that much weight.

How Important Is Aerobic Exercise in Shape Training?

Aerobic exercise helps strip away body fat to reveal your natural shape. Two aerobic workouts a week will give you fair results at best. But generally, it's preferable to perform four to five aerobic sessions a week, particularly if you want to shed body fat.

True, exercise does take more time per week with aerobics added in. But the rewards are greater. Case in point: At the Center for the Study of Nutrition and Metabolism in Boston, researchers divided 23 obese women into three groups: those who exercised 400 minutes a week (almost 7 hours) with aerobics and weights, those who worked out 200

minutes a week, and controls who did no exercise. All the women followed a calorie-controlled diet and stayed on the program for 12 weeks. The women who lost the most body fat were the ones in the 400-minute-a-week group. It all goes to show: Do more to lose more!

Will Shape Training Make My Muscles Sore?

You'll feel muscle soreness after starting a new routine, working out at a higher effort level, or doing a new exercise that stimulates muscles differently than exercises you've been using. If you feel sore every workout, you're probably exercising too hard. Cut back on the intensity and train at a more comfortable level until your body adjusts to the training load.

I'm Over Age 60. Can I Reshape Myself Too?

Remember the old advertising slogan, "You're not getting older, you're getting better"? That truism most definitely applies to women. Past menopause, your body starts secreting less estrogen. Male hormones, which exist in small amounts in a woman's body, start making up a slightly higher proportion of your hormone profile. One benefit of this is that it becomes easier for you to develop firm, body-shaping muscle, provided you exercise.

Also, according to research, people who exercise regularly tend to gain less body fat around and above the waist. Exercise is clearly a great hedge against upper-body fat and the diseases related to it.

One of the motivational barriers to regular exercise is the "I'm too old" excuse. Granted, anyone—regardless of age—should be checked out by a physician regularly, and definitely before starting an exercise program. With that caution in mind, mounds of research has proven the safety and effectiveness of exercise, particularly weight training, for senior adults.

Of course, many women past the age of 60 are already active, particularly when it comes to aerobic exercise. If you're one of them, adding weight training to your exercise routine multiplies the results. A recent study sheds some light on this: At San Diego State University, researchers selected 36 active women over age 60 to participate in a study. To be eligible, the women had to be aerobic exercisers who worked out at least three days a week and had been doing so for six months prior to the study.

Half the women were placed in an exercise group that performed weight training on machines three times a week; the other half formed the control group, who did no weight training at all. After six months, the weight-trained women increased their upper-body strength by as much as 65 percent. On average, they lost pounds of pure body fat and upped their lean muscle by slightly more than three pounds. There were no such changes among the controls.

The point is this: Regardless of how active you already are, you can get in even better shape by adding weight training to the exercise mix.

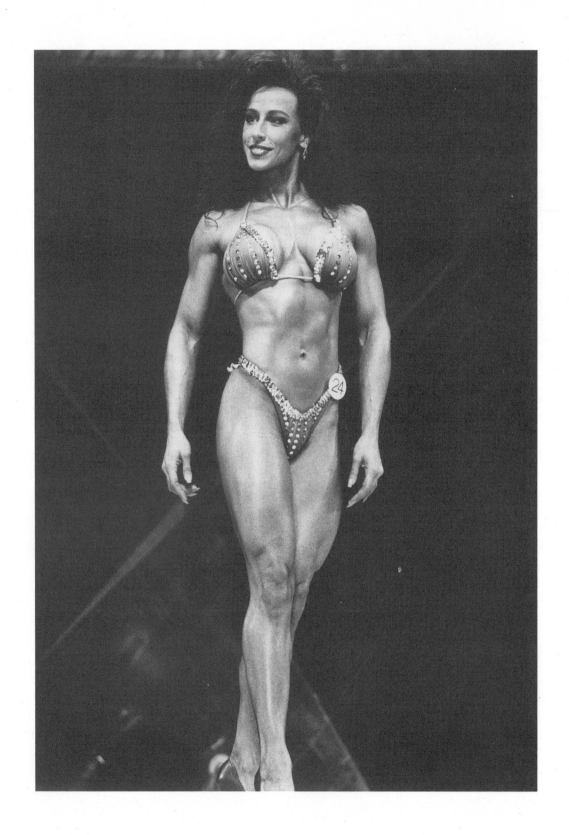

Shape-Training Aerobics

To get rid of unwanted fat, aerobic exercise is a must. It increases special fat-burning enzymes in the body, and it builds the number and density of tiny structures in cells called *mitochondria*, where fat and other nutrients are burned. The more mitochondria you have, the more fat your body can burn.

Aerobic exercise fights fat *during* exercise as well. In the first three to five minutes of aerobic exercise, your body starts burning mainly carbohydrate for fuel. After about 20 minutes, fat starts to kick in more fuel, especially as you pick up your pace. Furthermore, the more aerobically fit you are, the sooner your body switches over to fat stores and the greater percentage of fat you'll burn for fuel. An aerobically fit body is a fat-burning body.

How Can I Burn More Fat with Aerobic Exercise?

With aerobic exercise, try to gradually work up to a vigorous pace, or high intensity. Aerobic intensity is typically measured by *exercising heart rate*—how fast your heart beats while exercising. It's best to exercise at a level that's 65 to 85 percent of your maximum heart rate (MHR). To calculate your MHR, simply subtract your age from 220. Let's say you're 30 years old. Your MHR would be 190 (220 − 30). Your *target zone* would be 65 to 85 percent of that rate, or 124 (190 × .65) to 162 (190 × .85) beats per minute.

Exercising in the upper end of your zone will help you burn more fat. To help you find the upper end

Sherilyn Godreau keeps her body fat to a minimum with regular aerobics.

of your target zone, here are some examples:

Age	Maximum Heart Rate	85% of Maximum
20	200	170
25	195	166
30	190	162
35	185	157
40	180	153
45	175	149
50	170	145
55	165	140
60	160	136
65	155	132
70	150	128

To find your heart rate during exercise, take your pulse at the radial artery in either wrist or at the carotid artery. The radial artery is located near the center of the inside wrist. The carotid artery, which passes up the neck, is found just to the left or right of your windpipe.

Place your index and middle finger lightly over the artery. Don't press too hard, particularly on the carotid artery. Too much pressure can actually slow your pulse. Count the beats for 10 seconds, then multiply that number by six to get your heart rate for a minute.

An excellent indicator of your aerobic fitness is your heart rate at rest. In a very highly trained aerobic athlete, the heart rate is 30 to 40 beats a minute at rest; it is 70 to 80 beats a minute for normal people and 80 to 100 beats a minute for the sedentary and out-of-shape. Check your heart rate occasionally when you get up in the morning. If it's low, your heart is beating fewer times but pumping more blood with each beat. That means it's working more efficiently.

How Often Should I Do My Aerobics?

You can obtain fair results from two to three aerobic sessions a week. But as noted earlier, it's generally recognized that you'll make the best advances (especially in terms of fat loss) if you get aerobic exercise four to five days a week. Of course, frequency depends on your personal schedule. It's not always feasible to get in five aerobic sessions a week.

How Long Should I Work Out Aerobically?

The longer you do aerobics, the more fat you'll burn. After 20 minutes, your body starts relying more on fat for fuel, especially if you're working out in the upper end of your target zone. So for fat loss, you must try to work out aerobically for longer than 20 minutes. Also, for a conditioning effect on your heart, you need to exercise in your target heart rate zone for at least 20 minutes.

Is There a "Best" Time to Perform Aerobics for Fat Burning?

Any time you can fit intense, frequent aerobics into your schedule is the best time! For fat burning, however, some times—like first thing in the morning, before breakfast—are better than others. Pre-breakfast aerobics were first brought to the attention of fitness enthusiasts by *MuscleMag International* columnist John Parrillo, who uses it to get athletes in super-defined shape. According to Parrillo, the body is in a carbohydrate-deficient state in the morning. It has no choice but to start drawing on fat for energy as soon as you start exercising aerobically. Pre-breakfast aerobics also fire up your metabolism for the rest of the day, so the food you eat gets turned into energy, not stored as fat.

Parrillo also recommends performing aerobics after you work out with weights. Carbohydrate supplies the energy you need during your shape-training routine. But afterward, you have less carbohydrate available. Do your aerobics *after* your shape-training routine, and your primary fuel source then becomes fat—exactly what you want to burn.

There's more: Researchers have found that exercising aerobically between one and three hours after a meal burns up to 15 percent more calories than if you just plop down on the sofa after eating.

What Kind of Aerobics Should I Do?

It used to be that aerobics was aerobics was aerobics. Not anymore. Today there are special aerobics classes and new machines, which besides their primary heart-pumping action, provide muscle-toning stimulation to specific parts of the body. In each chapter, we recommend which aerobic exercises are best for improving your particular body type. However, the very best aerobics program is the one you enjoy—and will stick to.

No matter what type of aerobic activity you do, it should start with a warmup and finish with a cooldown. The warmup is five to ten minutes of light activity—walking at a slow pace, pedaling against very light resistance, slow stepping on a stair-climbing machine, and so forth. The warmup decreases stress on your heart, lowers your blood pressure, increases blood flow to your heart, and keeps your joints and muscles limber.

Similarly, a cooldown is five to ten minutes of less vigorous activity to help your heart rate return to normal. It also removes exercise-generated waste products from your muscles and keeps blood from pooling in your legs. If blood is allowed to collect in your legs, your blood pressure can drop sharply, possibly causing dizziness. The cooldown keeps blood circulating back toward the heart. Don't ever neglect either the warmup or the cooldown; make them essential parts of your aerobic workout.

After you've warmed up, you can choose from many forms of aerobics. These range from the conventional to the high-tech.

What Are the Conventional Aerobics Choices?

Even before *aerobic exercise* became a household word, people were doing it. The most popular conventional forms of aerobics are walking, jogging, running, bicycling, and swimming.

Walking

Millions of people walk for fitness, pleasure, or both. For aerobic exercise beginners, walking may be the best method of getting in shape. It's easy to do, convenient, and inexpensive. As for aerobic benefits, you can easily reach your target heart rate with brisk walking. Walking one mile burns approximately 100 calories.

If you're just starting a walking program, begin the first week by walking 20 minutes three times a week. For the next few weeks,

increase your time to 30 minutes. As you feel more energetic and fit, add an extra session or two to your weekly walking program. Try to work up to five sessions a week, for 30 to 45 minutes each time, especially if you're trying to pare off fat pounds. Remember to walk at a good clip, too, in order to keep your heart rate in its target zone. Here are some additional tips:

- Wear sturdy athletic shoes.
- Keep your head level as you walk, and look straight ahead.
- Bend your elbows at about a 90-degree angle, and keep them close to your sides. Swing your arms backward and forward as you walk.
- Let your heel strike the ground first, then roll from the heel to the ball of your foot. Push off with the ball of your foot for more momentum.
- Take long, smooth strides. Walk as briskly as you can. A good pace is $3\frac{1}{2}$ to 4 miles per hour.
- Breathe deeply but naturally as you walk.

Weighted Walking

A variation of walking is to use weights, which are strapped to your ankles, held in your hands, or worn on a belt and attached to your hips and chest. An advantage of weighted walking is that it's a great way to increase your intensity, particularly if you don't want to jog or run. In one study, researchers demonstrated that the intensity of walking at four miles per hour with ankle and hand weights was comparable to—and in some cases exceeded—that of running at five miles per hour. Weighted walking burned 120 to 158 calories a mile, whereas running expended 120 to 130 calories a mile.

It's best to begin a weighted walking program without weights, then add them later, starting with one-pound weights. Gradually increase the weight in one-pound increments until you're carrying about 5 to 10 percent of your body weight.

Racewalking

Another way to pick up the pace of walking without pounding the pavement by running is *racewalking*. Both a fitness pursuit and a competitive sport, racewalking is taking a series of steps in which one foot is kept in contact with the ground at all times, with the leg straight at the knee.

Compared to running, racewalking is less jarring on the body. Once you learn the racewalking technique, you can really move, at speeds between 4$\frac{1}{2}$ and 5$\frac{1}{2}$ miles per hour. That means you can burn more calories by racewalking than you can by walking. The faster you go, the faster the fat goes.

Mastering the racewalking moves takes a good bit of practice. Working with a qualified instructor

can help. Here are some guidelines to get you started:

- Bend your elbows to about 90 degrees, and let your arms swing freely.
- Keep your supporting leg straight. As that leg moves to the rear, keep its foot on the ground as long as you can before pushing off.
- Keep your hips loose so that they'll automatically shift to the straight leg. This will increase your stride length.
- Hit the ground heel first, pushing off from your back leg.
- Tilt your body forward slightly—about three to four inches—in a straight line.

Jogging and Running

If you've been walking but can't get your heart rate into the higher end of your zone, you may want to try jogging. The average speed for jogging is about five miles an hour. At higher speeds, you'll find it easier to run. A pace of six miles per hour or faster is running. Whether you jog or run, work on covering the same distance in less time. If you decide to run, increase your mileage by no more than 10 percent of the previous week's total. Here are some other pointers for jogging and running:

- Wear sturdy, well-cushioned running shoes.

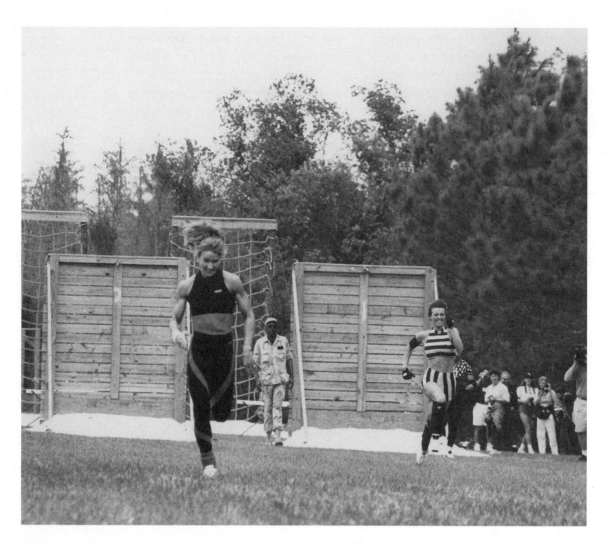

Jogging and running are great fat burners.

- Run in well-lit areas, and let people know your route.
- Run on smooth, well-cushioned tracks, rather than on hard pavement.
- Maintain good posture, with your head and chin up.
- Keep your elbows bent in a 90-degree angle and close to your side. Let your arms swing backward and forward as you jog or run.
- Take fairly short steps, letting your heel strike first.
- Breathe normally.
- Remember to take your pulse before, during, and after your run.

Biking

Outdoor biking is a great fat burner, expending as many as 500 calories an hour. Not only that, it tones up trouble spots like hips and thighs. But biking requires some skill to maneuver the bicycle safely and competently. If you haven't ridden recently, you'll have to do some practice riding to become familiar with your bike and the proper riding position.

To get the fitness benefits of biking, ride at a speed of 10 to 15 miles per hour on a straight stretch. Begin with about 20 minutes, two or three times the first week. Each week, gradually add to your distance and increase the frequency with which you ride. Don't ride on consecutive days, since your muscles (particularly your thigh muscles) need time to recover.

An outdoor cyclist must heed many safety precautions. Know the rules of the road, review bicycle safety, wear bright clothing, and always wear a bicycle helmet. Many communities have biking clubs; these are a good way to master this sport and meet other enthusiasts. Usually, biking shops have information on clubs and how to join them.

Swimming

If you like the water, swimming is pure fun. For people with joint problems, swimming is ideal for improving fitness without pain, since it's less jarring on the body than other forms of aerobics. The water displaces body weight, thus relieving stress on joints.

Swimming for fitness requires mastery of a few key strokes, namely the breaststroke, backstroke, and crawl. If you swim for aerobics, spend five to ten minutes swimming slowly to warm up. Swim at a comfortable pace, monitoring your pulse before, during, and after the workout. As with any aerobic program, start your swimming program gradually, adding laps weekly. Finish off your workout with slower swimming for a few minutes to cool down.

As enjoyable as swimming can be, it may not be your best bet for burning fat. One study comparing different types of aerobic exercise found that walkers and bikers lost weight, but swimmers actually gained weight. Other researchers have measured the body fat levels of aerobic athletes, only to find that swimmers don't lose as much fat as runners do. One possible explanation may be that water somehow causes the body to hang onto its fat as insulation against cold water temperatures.

Even so, swimming is a great way to start an aerobic exercise program, especially since it does improve aerobic fitness. But because swimming doesn't seem to burn fat very well, you may eventually want to check out other forms of aerobic exercise. However, swimming

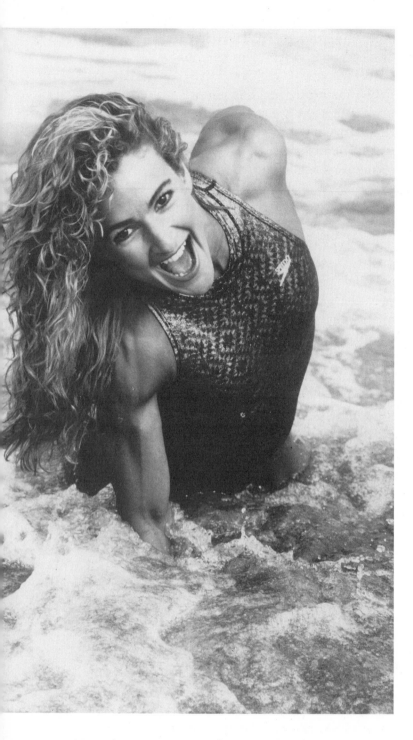

Not only are swimming and water exercise fun; they produce fitness benefits, too. (Model: Mia Finnegan)

remains a good option for I-frames, who want to conserve and build body mass.

What Kinds of Classes Provide Aerobic Exercise?

If you enjoy getting your exercise in a class setting, your basic choices are an aerobic dance class, bench stepping, and water exercise.

Aerobic Dance Classes

For millions of people, aerobic dance classes offer an enjoyable, effective way to get in shape. Since classes are intense and usually last an hour, you can maximize your fat-burning potential. Large muscle groups, particularly those of the lower body, are worked fairly hard, which improves muscle tone. As with most forms of aerobics, aerobic dancing at high intensities enhances your cardiovascular fitness. Plus, you achieve better coordination, posture, and body carriage, thanks to the often-intricate dance moves taught in classes.

The trend for a long time has been toward low-impact aerobic dancing. With this form of aerobics, at least one foot touches the floor throughout the aerobic portion of the workout. Dance steps are jumpless, knee lifts replace knee hops, and routines use large upper-body movements with a wide range of motion. Since low-impact aerobic dance eliminates the repetitive pounding on the joints on the dance floor, it is thought to be safer.

"Low impact" does not necessarily mean low intensity, however. Low-impact classes achieve intensity by increasing the amount of work done with the arms, the difficulty of the dance steps, and the cadence of those steps. Adding weights to the workout also increases intensity.

Low-impact aerobics does burn fat. One study looked into the effects of this type of workout on 15 sedentary women, ages 35 to 64. The women exercised for 10 weeks without changing or controlling their diets. On average, they lost 2.5 percent body fat.

Whatever class you choose, make sure the instructor is certified to teach aerobics. Also, see that your instructor works closely with you, according to your level of experience, to help you progress.

For convenience, you may opt to do aerobic dance at home with videos. There are hundreds to choose from, so before buying, rent a couple from your local video store or check out one from the library. Make sure the instructor's explanations are easy to understand and that the instructor is a good motivator. The workout should include a warmup, an aerobic segment at least 20 to 30 minutes long, and a cooldown. Also, you can tell a lot about the quality of the exercise program by the quality of the video production.

Bench Stepping

For greater aerobic fitness and muscle-toning action, many classes have added special benches to use with choreographed routines. As part of the routine, you step up and down on a bench. Benches come in various heights, typically ranging from 6 to 12 inches tall. Often, exercisers use handheld weights to increase the intensity of the effort and burn more calories.

In studies, bench stepping has stood up well as an aerobic exercise, burning more calories than walking. Exercise physiologists agree that it provides sufficient aerobic demand for both cardiovascular fitness and weight loss.

Water Exercise

In recent years, water exercise classes have grown in popularity at health clubs, rehabilitation centers, and hospitals. Water is an effective exercise medium because it offers a resistive, nonimpact environment for developing muscle tone, building strength, and enhancing cardiovascular fitness. Led by an instructor, you move vigorously against the resistance of the water to achieve these benefits.

Water exercise is best suited to people with arthritis, heart conditions, muscle problems, and debilitating injuries. But it's also beneficial if you're very overweight and want to gradually and safely start an exercise program.

One of the exercises used in these programs is *waterwalking,* or walking through water at midthigh depth. It's an excellent calorie burner—even better than walking on dry land! Research shows that waterwalking at about three miles per hour burns up twice as many calories as walking the same speed on land.

If you consider signing up for a water exercise class, make sure your instructor has a strong background in swimming, lifesaving, water safety, and CPR.

What Are Some High-Tech Approaches to Aerobics?

A number of machines are available to give you a high-tech aerobic workout. Some of these high-tech approaches that are worth checking out include Crossrobics, cross-country ski machines, stationary bikes, rowing machines, slide exercising, stair-climbing machines, and treadmills.

Crossrobics™
Without a doubt, the Crossrobics equipment (from Stairmaster) represents the "new generation" of training—one that combines aerobics and weight training into a single workout. The machine resembles a recumbent stair-climbing machine, but with a weight stack at your right. You can choose various programs, levels of intensity, and duration of exercise. A computerized readout of the program on a panel lets you see the upcoming peaks and valleys.

When the program begins, you push the pedals against resistance. This works your frontal thighs hard! The angled position of your body ensures that your thighs are directly isolated. As you work out, you must keep the weight stack suspended within a specific range. Depending on how you set up your Crossrobics program, the machine will ask you to increase your poundage on the weight stack about midway through the program for greater intensity.

With Crossrobics, you can pursue high-repetition training. This type of training has the potential to increase the number of mitochondria (cellular units that burn fat) in fast-twitch muscle fibers. With more mitochondria, muscle fibers burn more fat. Regular training on Crossrobics could turn your body into a fat-busting machine.

The day after using this machine for the first time, one of us (Maggie) felt leaner, as though fat had melted overnight. We foresee strength/aerobics machines of this ilk becoming staples in gyms everywhere.

Cross-Country Ski Machines

Few would argue that cross-country skiing is one of the best aerobic exercises ever. Years ago, innovative manufacturers developed cross-country ski machines, which are available for home use and in health clubs. Several types are on the market—some computerized—but all of the equipment places fitness-building demands on the lower and upper bodies.

With this equipment, you simulate the motion of a cross-country skier, alternating your arms and legs in a forward, then backward sliding motion. Some machines provide variability in speed and resistance for a wide range of exercise intensities.

Stationary Bicycles

One of the most popular high-tech forms of aerobics is using a stationary bicycle. It improves your fat-burning capability, increases your lower-body tone, and enhances your aerobic power, provided you exercise in the upper level of your target heart rate zone.

Sometimes boredom is a problem with stationary cycling. To counteract this, consider pedaling while watching television. Or make the ride more interesting by using some of the bike's motivating features, like computerized hill profiles, challenging resistance settings, or touch-screen readouts to monitor your progress.

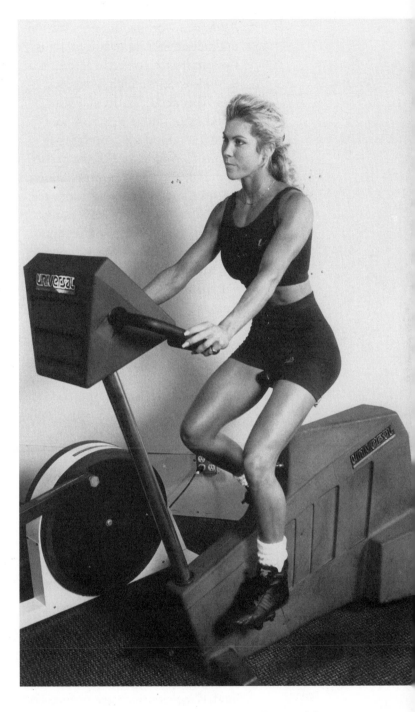

Stationary bicycles burn fat—and tone the thighs. (Model: Jennifer Goodwin)

When working out on a stationary bicycle, it's important to adjust the seat height correctly. If your seat is too low or too high, your legs won't pedal efficiently, and you could place undue stress on your knee joint. Find the correct seat height by placing one of the pedals in the fully lowered position. Sit on the bike and extend your leg to the pedal, making sure there's a slight bend in your knee. If not, readjust the seat accordingly.

Most stationary cycles have varying levels of difficulty. Initially, start at the lowest. Each week try to move up to the next level of difficulty. Be sure to take your heart rate before, during, and after your workout. Try to work out in your target heart range for at least 20 minutes.

Recumbent Stationary Bicycles

With a recumbent version of a stationary bike, you're seated so that your legs are parallel to the floor. Because you are in this position, the recumbent bike does a better job of isolating the thighs than a conventional stationary bike does. Once you start pedaling, practically all you feel is a leg-pumping burn.

Depending on the product, there's generous support for your hips, pelvis, and lower back, along with an extra-wide seat. Electronic models incorporate various levels of difficulty and intensity, giving you opportunities to do more each time you exercise.

Rowing Machines

One of the few devices that provide upper-body aerobic conditioning for your arms, back, torso, and midsection is the rowing machine. If you're skeptical about rowing machines, just take a look at the beautifully formed upper bodies of Olympic rowers! Also, recent studies have demonstrated that upper-body aerobic exercise is good for your heart.

Some rowing machines feature a screen that shows you "racing" against a pacer. The machine tells you how far behind or ahead you are, making the exercise almost like a video game.

Although your arms and back are worked the hardest, your legs get some action too, since you use them to push off with each stroke. Also, the rowing motion works the entire abdominal area. For a total aerobic workout, you might do half of your workout on a rowing machine, the other half on a stationary bike or stair-climbing machine.

Slide Exercising

For slide exercising, you stand on a flexible board slightly over six feet long with a special laminated surface. Simulating the motion of speed skating or roller skating, you actually slide on the device from side to side for a great lower-body workout. You'll glide best if you wear the "sliders" that fit over your athletic footwear and provide the right amount of friction for the exercise.

In university tests, the caloric cost of using this apparatus was found to be 20 percent greater than performing a standard aerobics workout and 16 percent higher than riding a stationary bicycle. A 10-minute workout on the slide expends 74 calories. To use up the same amount of calories while doing aerobics, you would have to exercise almost 13 minutes longer; while riding a stationary bike, you'd have to go about 12 minutes longer. In other words, you can burn more calories in less time, compared to other forms of aerobics.

Professional skaters have used this type of workout for years to condition their upper and lower bodies. Ideal for home aerobics use, the slide apparatus is available in sporting goods stores nationwide at a reasonable cost.

Stair-Climbing Machines

Like many mechanized aerobics machines, stair climbers provide instant feedback on calories burned, heart rate, and other variables. You can set the level of difficulty, too. These machines work the large muscles of the lower body, adding to the intensity of the effort. Leg strength can increase, too.

Research shows that stair-climbing machines do an excellent job of boosting aerobic power. In one study, 15 women between the ages of 25 and 48 worked out on a stair climber at moderately high intensities for 30 minutes three times a week for 12 weeks. After the study, their aerobic power had increased by 36 percent, an improvement that matches increases reported for walking, running, and cycling.

Experts advise that you work out on these machines in the lower end of your target heart rate zone. That's a little less than advised for other aerobic workouts, but these machines can overstress heart, lungs, and muscles if you push too hard. Plus, your muscles can fatigue too early, since the machine supplies resistance. If you fizzle out too early, you'll miss out on the fat-burning benefits of stair climbing.

Treadmills

Treadmills provide a great way to walk, jog, or run indoors, at home, or in a gym. You can adjust the speed of the treadmill according to your level of fitness, then increase the speed gradually as you become more conditioned. You can also adjust the grade or slope of the treadmill to make the exercise feel harder, as if you're jogging or running uphill. Some computerized treadmills let you choose certain programs in which the speed and grade automatically change while you're on the machine. Don't forget to monitor your heart rate.

To burn more calories, try swinging your arms while you walk on the treadmill. Research shows

You can walk, jog, or run on a treadmill. (Model: Jennifer Goodwin)

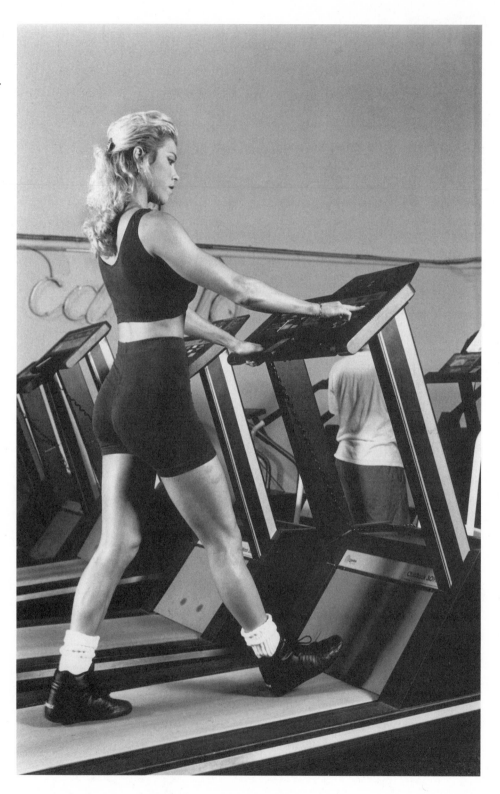

that vigorous arm swinging increases your calorie-burning potential by 50 percent. It also gives your upper body a good workout.

How Can I Add Variety to My Aerobics Routine?

One way to stay motivated in your aerobic exercise program is to combine various types of aerobics using a "cross-training" approach. For example, you might try this routine:

- 5 minutes of walking around an indoor track (warmup)

- 10 to 15 minutes on a stair-climbing machine
- 10 to 15 minutes on a rowing machine
- 10 to 15 minutes on a stationary bicycle
- 5 minutes of walking around an indoor track (cooldown)

You can experiment with other combinations, too.

Whatever aerobic activity you pursue, be sure to keep track of your heart rate and the duration and frequency of your workouts. That way, you can ensure you're making steady progress.

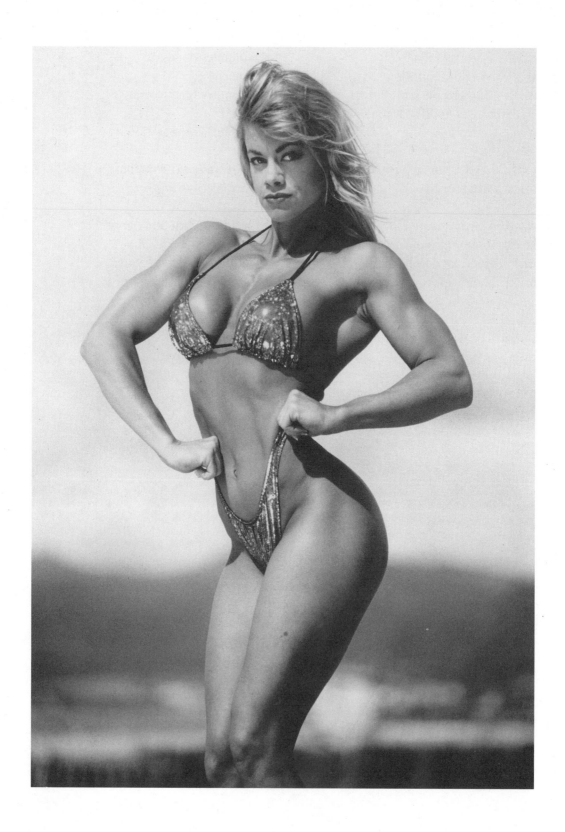

6

The A-Frame: Sculpting Legs and Hips

Do you hate the size of your hips and thighs? Are they sizable where they should be sleek? Have you given up on ever seeing leg-firming muscle underneath all the padding?

If you answered yes to even one question, don't give up just yet. Those saddlebags may not be as immovable as you think. Out-of-shape thighs and hips can become lean through shape training, which tightens those areas right up.

It's really important to be selective about the exercises you do. The shape-training routine for A-frames includes *compound exercises*. These work several muscles at once and develop muscle tone and strength.

In addition to the compound exercises, this routine features two or three *isolation exercises,* which target certain muscles or parts of muscles and are excellent for firming hard-to-reach areas. Most of your lower-body exercises will be in the moderate- to high-repetition range—perfect for toning and trimming.

Many women with A-frames obsess over working the thighs and hips, to the point of neglecting other body parts. But reshaping an A-frame involves looking at the body as a whole, not just its lower portions. As an A-frame, you need to spend equal time on developing your shoulders, back, and chest. That way, you can offset your wider hips, creating more balanced proportions. To do that, you'll perform exercises for your upper body using heavier poundages and low repetitions. These will develop your upper body in proportion to your lower, but without adding bulk.

Marla Duncan has near-perfect proportions.

Shape-Training Exercises for A-Frames: Thighs and Buttocks

First, let's look at the exercises aimed at trimming and toning your lower body.

Wide-Stance Barbell Squat
Targets: Inner thighs and buttocks

The barbell squat develops the entire lower body, including the thighs, hamstrings, hip muscles, and calves. To do this exercise, it's wise to follow these guidelines:

- *Wear the proper attire.* Since the bar will be situated across your neck, wear a T-shirt rather than a leotard or tank top. The shirt will

Wide-stance barbell squat

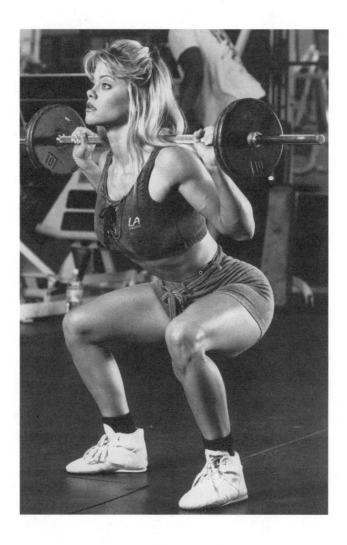

protect your neck and alleviate any discomfort.

- *Set the squat rack at the proper height.* Squats are usually performed with a *squat rack*. This is a cagelike device with adjustable hooks at each end that hold the barbell in place. You can change the height of the barbell by adjusting the placement of the hooks.

  The correct height of the barbell on the rack should be slightly below shoulder level. If the barbell is too high, you'll have to stand on your toes to remove it from the rack, and this is a dangerous maneuver.

  The rack should also have *catchers* at each end—bars located near the bottom of the rack to catch the barbell in case you should fail to complete the lift.

  As you get ready to do a set, lift the bar off the rack, then rerack it when you've completed your set.

- *Wear a lifting belt.* A sturdy lifting belt, tightly secured around your waist, is an excellent way to stabilize your back and help you do the exercise with better form, especially since you'll be attempting fairly heavy poundages.

- *Breathe naturally.* While performing squats, it's very important not to hold your breath. Breathing correctly during this exercise means breathing naturally.

- *Warm up properly.* Always begin your set of squats with a light warmup, using an unloaded bar. Try to do 12 to 15 repetitions in preparation for your heavier sets.

- *Consider using a spotter.* A *spotter* is someone who knows the exercise well enough to coach you through its correct performance. Until you become more experienced in performing this exercise, it's a good idea to work with a spotter to ensure that you're squatting correctly and safely. Once you get the feel of it, you'll find that the squat is a very easy and comfortable exercise to do.

To begin the exercise, place a barbell behind your neck and hold it with your hands placed about shoulders' width apart. Your feet should be about 22 to 24 inches apart, with your toes pointed outward. Keep your head up and your back as straight as possible. Lower your body slowly, until the tops of your thighs are parallel to the floor. Do not go any lower. Using the strength of your thighs, press back up slowly to the starting position. At the top of the movement, squeeze your buttocks together tightly to activate the gluteal muscles of the hip.

After you have warmed up by using an unloaded bar, gradually add weight, about five pounds at a time. Keep your repetitions fairly high (12 to 15), since your goal is toning, not building.

Close-Stance Hack Squat
Targets: Outer thighs

A close-stance hack squat is performed on a special machine called a *hack slide*, a popular piece of equipment in most gyms and health clubs. Step into the machine and face forward. Place your feet a few inches apart, with your toes pointing forward. Release the safety latches, and slide up and down by bending and straightening your knees. In the bent-knee position, your thighs should be parallel with the platform of the machine.

Close-stance hack squat

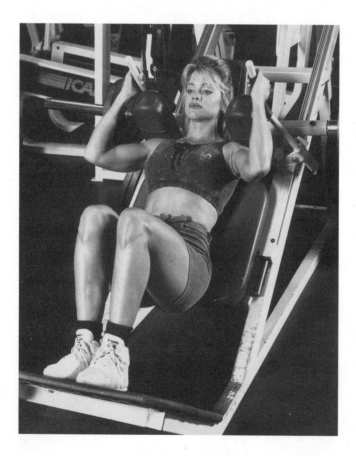

Pulley Leg Curl
Targets: Hamstrings and buttocks

Attach an ankle strap to your right ankle, and hook that strap to a lower-pulley machine. Lie face-down on a bench placed perpendicular to the pulley machine. Make sure there's enough room between the bench and the machine that you can lift and lower the selected weight.

Curl your right leg up slowly until your calf touches the back of your upper thigh (your leg biceps). Return to the starting position and repeat the exercise for the suggested number of repetitions. Repeat the exercise with your left leg.

Dumbbell Bun Burner
Targets: Buttocks

The dumbbell bun burner is a terrific bun tightener. Place two dumbbells on the floor about 12 to 18 inches apart. Stand with your legs comfortably apart. Slowly bend over, keeping a slight arch in your back. Try to keep your legs straight, although you may have to bend your knees slightly. As you bend over, get a good stretch in the back of your legs. At the bottom of the movement, pick up the dumbbells and slowly return to an erect position. While lifting the weights, use the strength of your hips and thighs, not your back. Throughout this portion of the

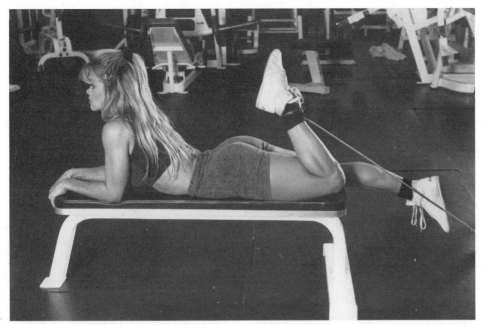

Pulley leg curl

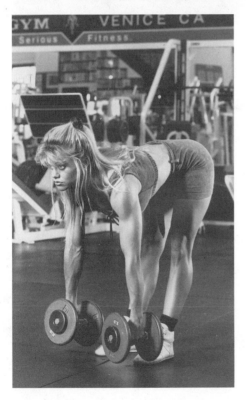

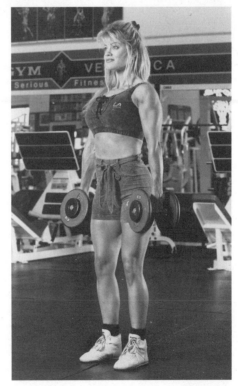

Dumbbell bun burner

exercise, squeeze your buttocks together as hard as possible until you're fully erect.

You can also perform this exercise with a barbell.

Do-Anywhere Bun Burner
Targets: Buttocks

Demonstrating the A-frame exercises in this chapter is Marla Duncan, a Ms. Fitness winner and columnist for *MuscleMag International*. Marla is known for her shapely proportions, particularly her lower body. Here's one of her secrets: She works the gluteal muscles of her buttocks all day long by contracting those muscles while seated at work, home, or in her car. You can do the same, and no one will even know!

Shape-Training Exercises for A-Frames: Upper Body

Your second shape-training goal is to build your upper body, particularly your shoulders. Shapely shoulders, toned through weight training, help offset a large hipline. By adding some muscle and a little more width to your shoulders, shape training will make your hips and waist appear smaller and more proportionate with the rest of your body. It's all a part of the illusion shape training creates in your figure.

But don't worry about turning into a he-man. Ninety-nine percent of the female population simply can't develop hulky muscles. Women don't have the hormones to do it. You can, however, take your figure to its optimum physical shape with the exercises that follow.

These exercises are an effective way to better endow your shoulder line. Incorporated into your overall shape-training routine, they promise to sculpt your shoulders and upper body into better shape in only a few short weeks. Additionally, with an improved shoulder line, your posture will look better and appear more graceful.

Dumbbell Overhead Press
Targets: Front and outer shoulders

Sit on a bench and grasp a dumbbell in each hand, palms facing forward. Place the weights at shoulder level, then press them upward to an overhead position. Lock your elbows at the top of the movement. Slowly lower the dumbbells to the shoulder-level position. Repeat the exercise for the suggested number of repetitions.

Bench Side Lateral Raise
Targets: Rear shoulders

Take a face-forward position on an incline bench. Hold a dumbbell in each hand, with your palms facing down. Keeping your arms

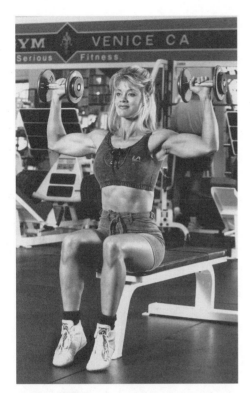

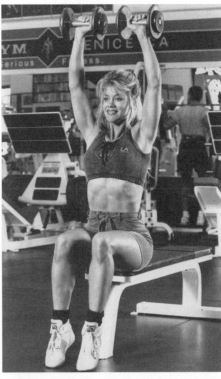

Dumbbell overhead press

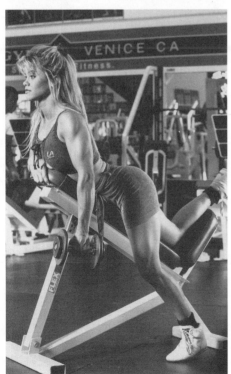

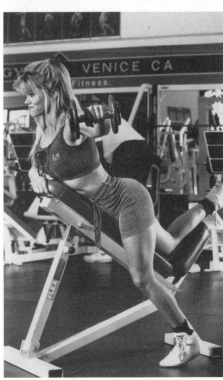

Bench side lateral raise

straight and your elbows locked, raise your right arm up in an arc to an overhead position. Lower the weight slowly, and repeat with the other arm. Continue alternating each arm in this fashion for the suggested number of repetitions.

Upright Row
Targets: Tops of shoulders

Grasp a barbell with your hands about shoulders' width apart. Keeping the bar close to your body, lift it to a position just above your shoulders. Lower slowly to the starting position. Repeat the exercise for the suggested number of repetitions.

Machine Chin-Up
Targets: Upper back and biceps

Designed to build the muscles of the upper back, machine chin-ups are a high-tech version of the traditional chin-up, in which you hoist yourself up to a bar. Traditional chin-ups are very difficult for women to perform because of their naturally weaker upper bodies. Machine chin-ups are a much better alternative. Depending on the brand, the machines for this exercise counterbalance your weight in some way so you can perform the exercise with assistance from the machine.

To begin, select a weight that's comfortable, usually 10 to 20 per-

Upright row

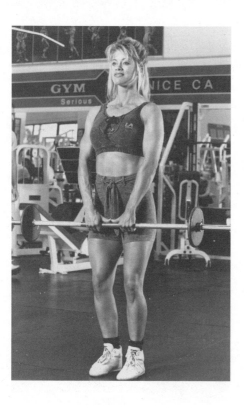

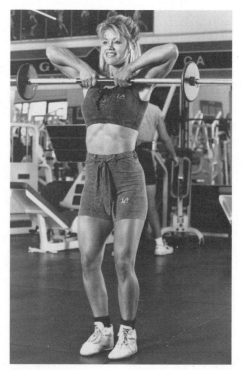

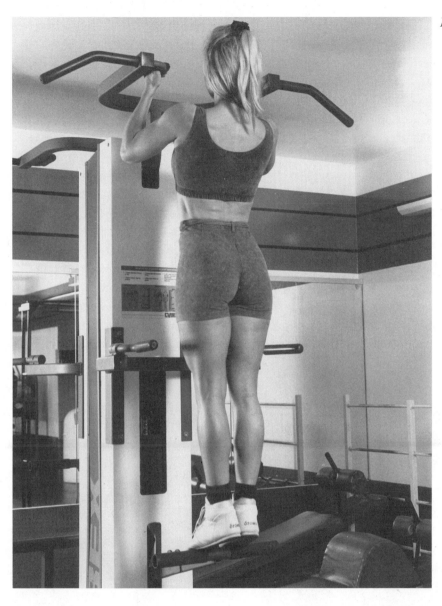

Machine chin-up

cent lighter than your present body weight. You may have to experiment on a few repetitions. Step on the platform and grab the upper bar. As you pull yourself up, the platform will move up with you, giving you the nudge you need to complete your reps. With each set, decrease the weight you select so that you're lifting more of your own body weight. With time, you'll be able to perform chin-ups on your own, without the machine's assistance.

Close-Grip Front Pulldown
Targets: Upper back

To perform the close-grip front pull-down, you use a pulley machine. Take a close grip on the bar, with your hands placed several inches apart and palms facing toward you. Pull the bar straight down in front of your body, so that it touches your upper chest. Slowly return it to the top position, and repeat the exercise.

Dumbbell Bench Press
Targets: Pectoral (chest) muscles

Although it will not increase or decrease the size of your breasts, the dumbbell bench press will solve two figure problems: a "flat" chest and sagging breasts. It does this by building up your pectoral muscles, the muscular foundation upon which your breasts lie. On flat-chested figures, the result is a muscular cleavage that looks alluring. For a larger-breasted woman whose breasts sag, the bench press firms the muscles underneath the bosom to create a lifted appearance.

Lie back on a flat exercise bench and hold a dumbbell in each hand. Your palms should face in the direction of your feet. Position the dumbbells at the sides of your chest. From this point, press the dumbbells

Close-grip front pulldown

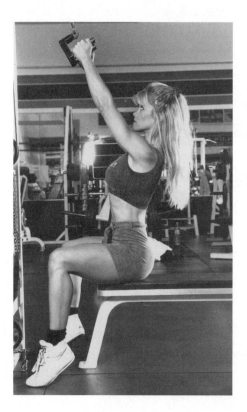

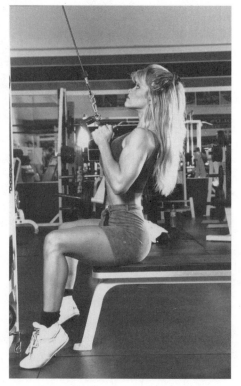

SHAPE TRAINING

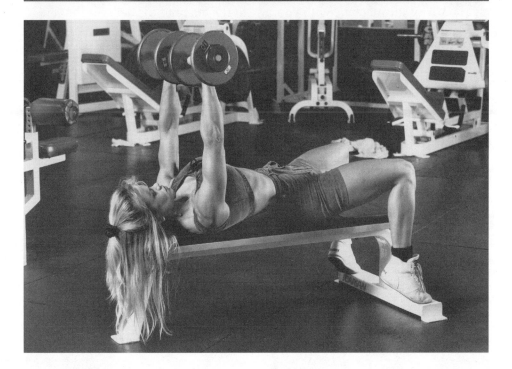

Dumbbell bench press

up to a position just above your chest. Lock your elbows out at the top. Slowly lower the dumbbells to the starting position. Repeat the exercise for the suggested number of repetitions.

Machine Curl
Targets: Biceps of arm

Sit in the arm-curl machine and grasp the handles or bar, depending on the type of equipment. Curl your arms upward in an arclike motion, squeezing at the top of the exercise. Return to the start position and repeat.

Triceps Pressdown
Targets: Triceps (muscles at rear of arm)

You do the triceps pressdown on a high-pulley machine. Start by grasping the bar of the machine with your hands about eight inches apart. Press down until your arms are perfectly straight and elbows locked tightly.

Try to keep your elbows at your sides during the exercise. Slowly return to the starting position. Repeat the exercise.

Twisting Crunch
Targets: Side and front abdominals

Lie on your back, and drape your lower legs over a bench. Place your hands behind your head. Using the strength of your abdominal muscles, bring your torso up toward your knees, but not all the way up. Twist to the right slightly, then return to the starting position. On the next repetition, twist to the left. Alternate in this manner throughout the set.

Twisting Leg Raise
Targets: Lower and side abdominals

Machine curl

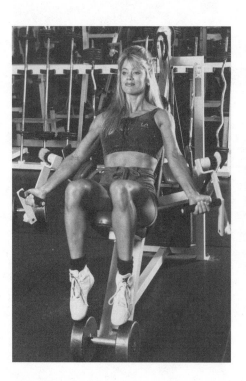

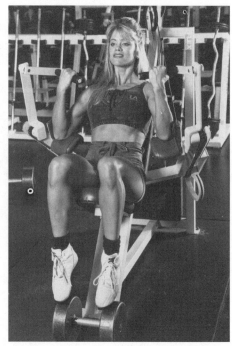

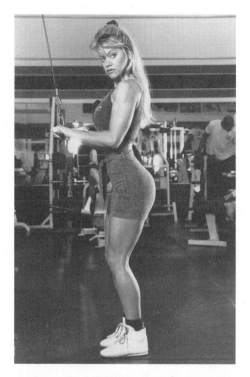

To do the twisting leg raise, you'll need a dip stand or similar apparatus in which you can support yourself between two parallel bars. Facing away from the equipment, hoist yourself up so that your legs

Twisting crunch

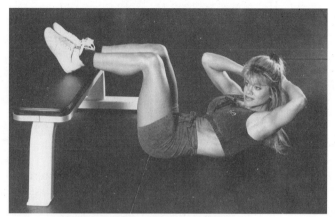

Triceps pressdown

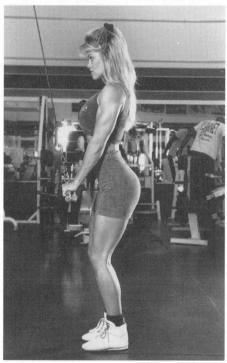

Twisting leg raise

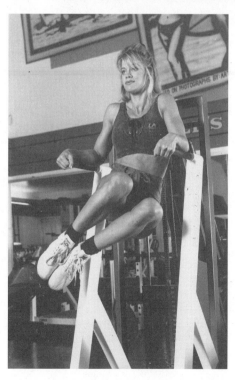

cannot touch the floor. Brace yourself on the stand with your lower arms. With your legs together, bend your knees and raise them so that your upper thighs are parallel to the floor and your lower legs are vertical to the floor. As you do this, twist your body and legs to the right. Repeat this action to the left. Continue alternating in this manner throughout the set.

The Shape-Training Routine for A-Frames

Your routine is a four-day split routine in which you exercise your upper body on Monday and Thursday and your lower body on Tuesday and Friday. Following each routine, try to perform the recommended aerobics for fat burning. Wednesday and Sunday have been

Shape-Training Routine: A-Frames

MONDAY/THURSDAY

Emphasis:	Upper-body development with shoulder specialization
Warmup:	5–10 minutes of relaxed walking
Exercise style:	Heavy weights and low repetitions (6–10)

Routine

Exercise*	Sets**	Repetitions
Dumbbell overhead press	Warmup set (light weight)	10–12
	3 (increase poundage each set)	6–10
Bench side lateral raise	Warmup set (light weight)	10–12
	3 (increase poundage each set)	6–10
Upright row	Warmup set (light weight)	10–12
	3 (increase poundage each set)	6–10
Machine chin-up	Warmup set (light weight)	10–12
	3 (increase poundage each set)	6–10
Close-grip front pulldown	Warmup set (light weight)	10–12
	3 (increase poundage each set)	6–10
Dumbbell bench press	Warmup set (light weight)	10–12
	3 (increase poundage each set)	6–10
Machine curl	Warmup set (light weight)	10–12
	3 (increase poundage each set)	6–10
Triceps pressdown	Warmup set (light weight)	10–12
	3 (increase poundage each set)	6–10

Aerobics

Follow the above exercise routine with 30–45 minutes of bench-stepping aerobics, Crossrobics, cross-country ski machine exercise, recumbent stationary cycling, slide exercising, or stair-climbing machine.

designated as rest days; however, you could also use these days to do aerobics, if you prefer. For a fifth session of aerobics, we recommend that you set aside a Saturday workout for aerobics only. The more aerobic workouts you can get in, the more fat you'll burn.

TUESDAY/FRIDAY

Emphasis:	Lower-body toning
Warmup:	5–10 minutes of relaxed walking
Exercise style:	Moderate weights and high repetitions (12–15)

Routine

Exercise*	Sets**	Repetitions
Wide-stance barbell squat	Warmup set (light weight)	10–12
	3 (increase poundage each set)	12–15
Close-stance hack squat	Warmup set (light weight)	10–12
	3 (increase poundage each set)	12–15
Pulley leg curl	Warmup set (light weight)	10–12
	3 (increase poundage each set)	12–15
Dumbbell bun burner	Warmup set (light weight)	10–12
	3 (increase poundage each set)	12–15
Twisting crunch	1	As many as possible (at least 25)
Twisting leg raise	1	As many as possible (at least 25)

Aerobics

Follow the above exercise routine with 20–30 minutes of fast walking.

WEDNESDAY/SUNDAY

Rest

SATURDAY

Emphasis:	Fat burning

Aerobics

Warm up with 5 minutes of relaxed walking. Cross-train for 30–45 minutes in the following manner: 10–15 minutes on a recumbent stationary bicycle, 10–15 minutes on a rowing machine, and 10–15 minutes on a cross-country ski machine, stair-climbing machine, or Crossrobics machine. Be sure to cool down with some relaxed walking. If you don't have access to this equipment, perform some conventional aerobics, such as weighted walking, racewalking, jogging, or running.

*If your gym or workout facility does not have certain types of machines or equipment, refer to Appendix C for exercise substitutions.

**If you've never worked out with weights before, perform just 3 sets (1 warmup set and 2 regular sets).

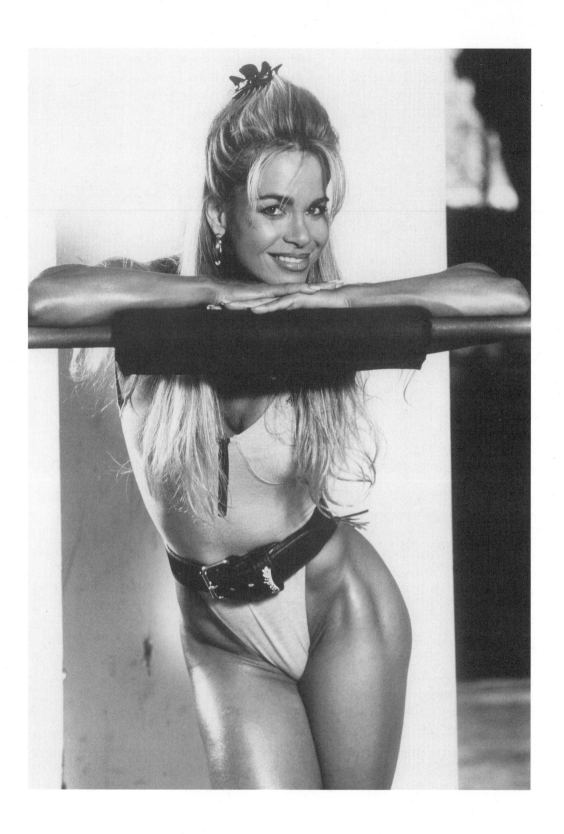

The H-Frame: Whittling Away Your Waist

You're endowed with a solidly built, athletic shape. That's a plus, since it means you're blessed with healthy muscle to keep your bones strong and your body fit. As for shape, your upper and lower bodies are of relatively equal proportion. The trouble is right smack dab in the middle—your tummy. You may need to trim some fat off your waist, tone your abdominal muscles back into shape, or both.

A lot of people believe that the way to a lean, fat-free waistline is doing hundreds of ab exercises every day. That's only part of the solution. True, waistline exercises will firm up abdominal muscles underneath the fat and wake up sluggish circulation so fat burning can proceed. The best and fastest plan of attack is to follow a low-fat diet, do plenty of aerobic exercise each week, and perform the right abdominal exercises to make you look as trim as you can be.

Exercise and diet will transform your H-frame into the more desirable hourglass look. But good looks aren't the only benefit. The four sets of muscles that make up your abdominal column work together with your back muscles to help you sit straight, stand tall, and move with ease. If you've ever had a lower-back problem, you know that one of the first rules in restoring health and preventing future back ailments is to strengthen your ab muscles.

Remember this, too: Trimming that roll around the middle lowers your risk factor for heart disease, high blood pressure, diabetes, some cancers, and many other

Amy Fadhli has a pleasing athletic shape.

life-shortening diseases. There's a healthy payoff for anyone—not just H-frames—who gives the abdominals individual attention.

How Does Diet Improve One's Waistline?

Cutting fatty foods from your daily diet should be part of a total plan to zap tummy fat. Interestingly, when a group of 124 women reduced dietary fat, they each lost 10 to 15 pounds, and more than half the women lost body fat mostly from their abdomen.

Sugar-laden foods are a no-no as well. When your body gets too much sugar at once, it releases lots of the hormone insulin. Insulin stimulates fat cells to open up so fat can come in and be stored. So cut out soft drinks, chocolate, and other sweets. If you don't notice some difference early on, reduce foods like breads and pastas and stick to more natural carbohydrates like potatoes and whole-grain cereals. Make dietary changes gradually, or else you're more likely to blow your diet. For more advice on diet, see Chapter 13.

Be forewarned about dieting: Going on and off a reducing diet can make your waistline look like the equator. The proof is in some interesting research conducted at Yale University several years ago. Researchers there studied pre-menopausal women who had gone up and down in weight many times during their lives—a result of repeated efforts at dieting. What they found was intriguing: Women with a history of on-again, off-again dieting and fluctuations in weight tended to gain fat mostly in the abdominal region. In other words, when fat returns after you go off a diet, it returns to your waistline. So don't diet too drastically, but rather follow a healthy nutritional plan you can stick to.

Breakthrough News: Some Aerobic Exercise Can Spot-Reduce the Waistline

Researchers at the Washington University School of Medicine in St. Louis, Missouri, put a group of men and women aged 60 to 70 on a 9- to 12-month exercise program that consisted of walking or jogging. On average, the subjects exercised 45 minutes several times a week. By the end of the study, both the men and the women had lost weight. But get this: Most of their weight was shed from the abdominal area. This all goes to show that a simple exercise program like walking or jogging can melt off abdominal fat, which creeps on as we get older. From a health perspective, this type of exercise—fighting waistline flab—may reduce the risk of diseases linked to abdominal fat.

Compared to other fat storage sites on the body, the abdominal region is *lipolytically active*. This means it gives up fat easily. One of the best ways to activate this process is aerobic exercise. A group of Canadian researchers put this to the test. In their study, 13 obese women exercised moderately for 90 minutes four or five times a week for 14 months. At the end of the study, the women underwent CT scans to detect any changes in body fat patterning. More flab was lost from the abdominal region than from the midthigh, proving that ab fat is easily burned with a consistent, long-term exercise program.

Based on this information, the best flab-busting aerobics for your midsection include walking, jogging or running, and treadmill exercise. For best results, you should try to perform aerobics five times a week.

Shape-Training Exercises for H-Frames

Your shape-training routine concentrates on overall body development, toning, and strengthening, along with a midsection specialization program to help you deflate your "spare tire." You'll perform your core routine on Monday and Friday and your midsection routine on Wednesday and Saturday. Shape-training aerobics are included for fat

burning. What follows are the exercises you'll perform in your routine.

Dumbbell Lunge to the Front
Targets: Thighs, buttocks, and hamstrings

Lunges are an excellent shaping and toning exercise for the lower body. To begin, hold a dumbbell in each hand at your sides. While keeping your back straight, step forward on your right leg as far as possible until your right thigh is parallel to the floor. Try to hold your left leg as straight as possible. From this point, step back to the starting position. Continue the exercise on the right leg for the suggested number of repetitions, then repeat the exercise on the left leg.

You can also do this exercise with a barbell draped across your rear shoulders.

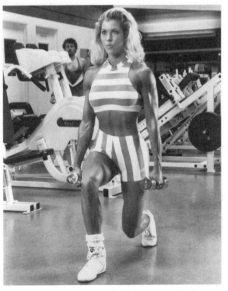

Dumbbell lunge to the front

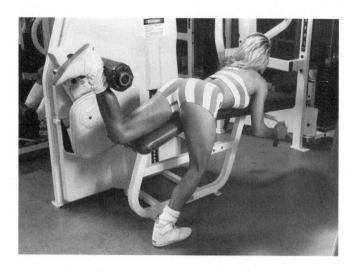

Single-leg curl

Single-Leg Curl
Targets: Hamstrings and buttocks

Lie facedown on the leg curl bench. Hook the rear of your lower right leg to the padded roller. Curl your leg up in an arc as far as you can. Continue the exercise for the suggested number of repetitions, then work the left leg in the same manner.

Reverse Hyperextension
Targets: Buttocks

To do reverse hyperextensions, you'll need a bench designed especially for this exercise. Lie face forward on the hyperextension bench so that your torso extends off the front of the bench and your pelvis is braced by the pads. Your legs should be secured behind you. With your hands behind your head, bend forward at the waist as far as you can. Squeeze your buttocks together, and use their strength to lift your torso back up in an arc to the starting position. Perform between 25 and 50 repetitions. Try to keep your buttocks contracted throughout the exercise.

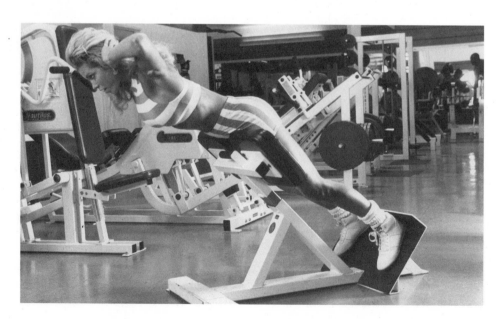

Reverse hyperextension

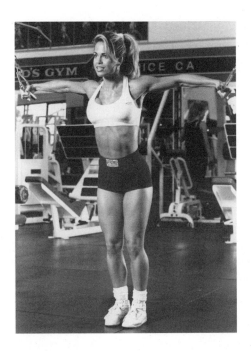

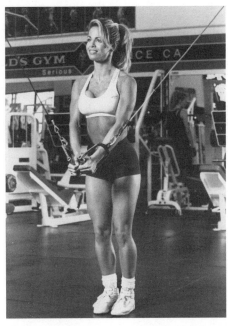

Cable crossover

Cable Crossover
Targets: Pectoral (chest) muscles

Stand between two cable stations, and take a pulley handle in each hand. Lean slightly forward, and bring your elbows together in front of your body. In this contracted position, squeeze your pectoral (chest) muscles hard. Slowly return the pulleys to the starting position, and repeat the exercise for the suggested number of repetitions.

Machine Shoulder Press
Targets: Shoulders

Sit in the shoulder-press machine facing forward, and take hold of the handles (or bar) with your palms facing forward. Press the handles up to an overhead position. Lock

your elbows at the top. Lower slowly. Repeat the exercise for the suggested number of repetitions.

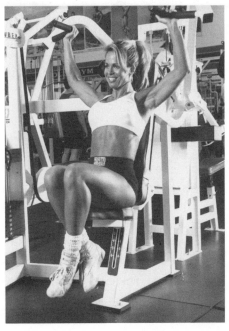

Machine shoulder press

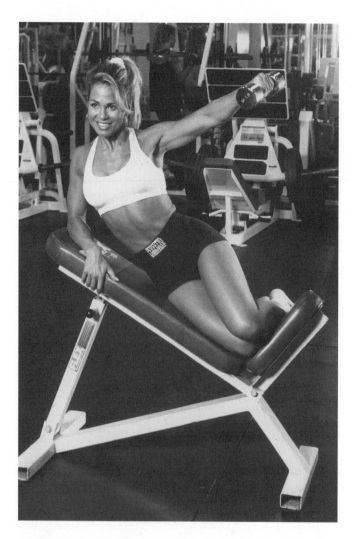

Incline side lateral raise

Keeping the dumbbell to the side and your arm straight, lift the weight to a position slightly higher than shoulder level. Slowly return to the starting position, and continue the exercise for the suggested number of repetitions. Repeat the exercise with the left arm.

Low Seated Pulley Row
Targets: Upper Back

Perform the low seated pulley row on a cable machine with a low pulley. Sit on the floor or a low bench in front of the machine, and grasp the pulley handle. Pull the handle horizontally into your midsection. Hold this position for a second or two, then slowly let your arms straighten out to stretch your upper back muscles. Pull in again, and repeat the exercise for the suggested number of repetitions.

Concentration Curl
Targets: Biceps of arms

Grasp a dumbbell in your right hand, and sit at the end of a flat exercise bench. Rest your right elbow against the inside of your thigh, and begin with your right arm straight. Flex your elbow, curling up toward your upper arm. Slowly return to the starting position, and repeat the exercise for the suggested number of repetitions.

Repeat the exercise with the left arm.

Incline Side Lateral Raise
Targets: Shoulders

A nice shaping exercise for your outer shoulders is the incline side lateral raise. Lie sideways on a full-length incline bench. Hold a dumbbell in your right hand at your thigh, with your palm facing your thigh.

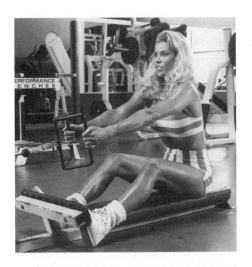

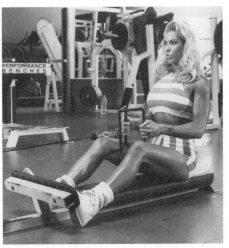

*Low seated
pulley row*

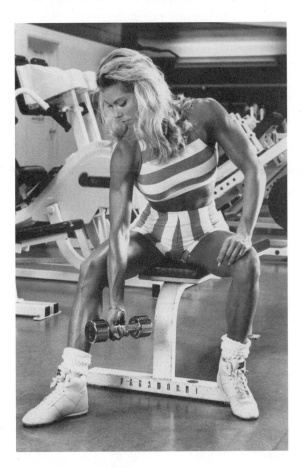

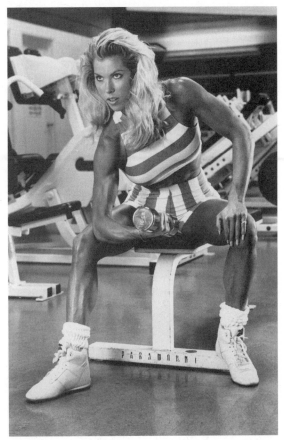

Concentration curl

Machine Dip
Targets: Triceps (back of upper arms)

A dip machine counterbalances your weight to help you perform the exercise. Step on the platform and hold on to the bars at your side. Begin with your arms straight. Then bend your elbows and lower your body as far as you can. Lift yourself back up to the starting position. As you lift yourself up, the platform will move up with you, assisting you in the exercise.

With each set, decrease the weight you select. Perform as many repetitions as you can.

Machine dip

Low-Pulley Triceps Extension
Targets: Triceps (back of upper arms)

Kneel on the floor, with your back to the cable machine. Hold onto the pulley handle (a short, straight bar handle is best) with your palms facing up and your elbows bent. Your upper arms should be pressed close to your head. Extend your arms up to a position nearly perpendicular to the floor, and lock your elbows out. Lower slowly to the starting position. Repeat the exercise for the suggested number of repetitions.

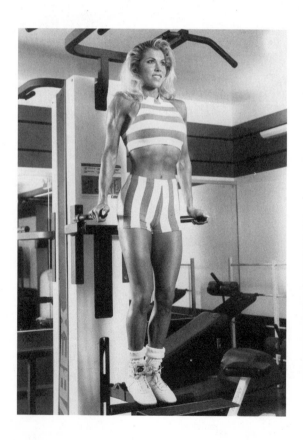

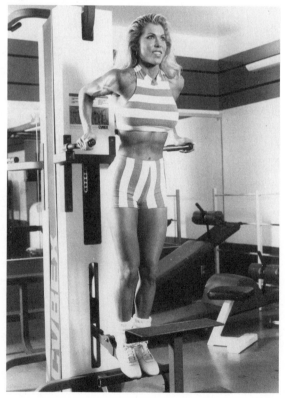

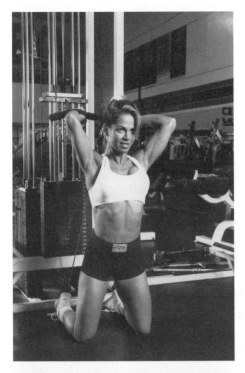

Midsection Specialization Exercises

The following shape-training exercises will give you a slimmer profile by tightening and toning up your abdominal muscles. Strong ab muscles burn more calories even at rest and can therefore help prevent your belly bulge from returning.

Decline Bench Crunch

The decline bench crunch is an abdominal toner performed on a decline bench. Lie back on the bench with your knees bent and your feet secured at the foot of the bench. Place your hands behind your head with your elbows out. Using the strength of your abdominal muscles, bend at the waist and bring your upper body toward your knees, but not all the way up. Repeat the exercise for as many repetitions as you can.

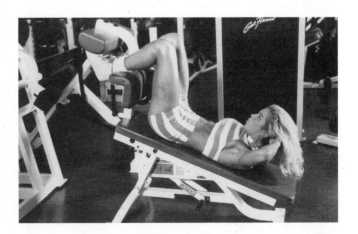

Low-pulley triceps extension

Decline bench crunch

Side Crunch

The side crunch is an excellent waist trimmer. Lie on your side on a flat bench so that your torso extends off the bench at the waist and is free to move up and down. Have someone secure your feet at the other end of the bench. Place your hands behind your head with your elbows out. Bend at the waist, slowly lowering and raising your torso. Perform as many repetitions as you can.

Side crunch

Repeat the exercise on the other side.

Knee-Up

To do knee-ups, you'll need a dip stand. Facing away from the stand, hoist yourself up between the two parallel dipping bars and support yourself there with your legs straight. Bend your knees and pull your thighs in toward your midsection. Return to the starting position

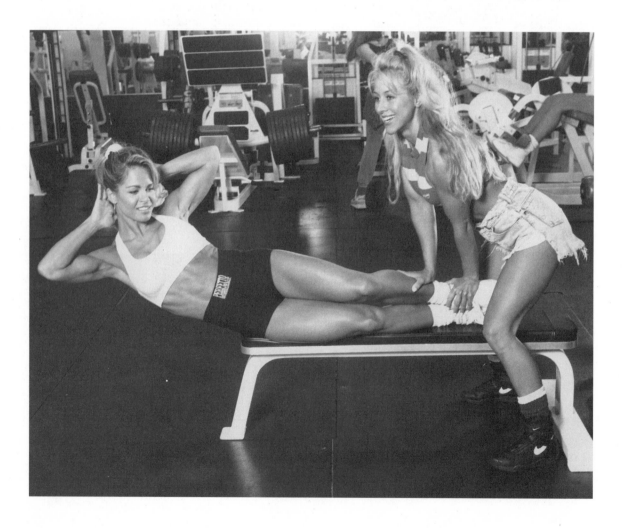

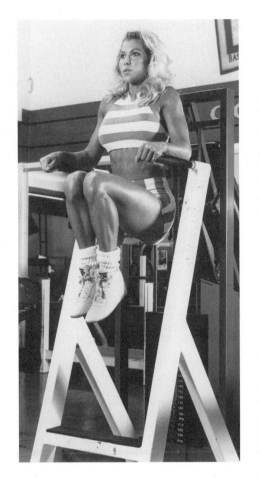

Knee-up

and repeat. Perform as many repetitions as you can.

Dumbbell Side Bend
Take a dumbbell in each hand, and hold them at your sides. Stand with your feet about a foot apart. Bend at your waist to the side, first to the right, then to the left, stretching as far as you can. Continue bending this way for as many reps as you can do.

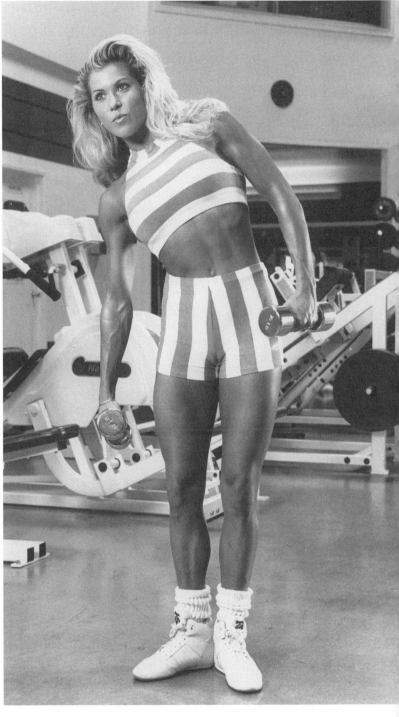

Dumbbell side bend

Shape-Training Routine: H-Frames

MONDAY/FRIDAY

Emphasis:	Lower- and upper-body toning and strengthening
Warmup:	5–10 minutes of relaxed walking
Exercise style:	Moderate to high poundages and medium reps (12–15)

Routine

Exercise*	Sets	Repetitions
Dumbbell lunge to the front	Warmup set (light weight)	10–12
	2–3 (increase poundage each set)	12–15
Single-leg curl	Warmup set (light weight)	10–12
	2–3 (increase poundage each set)	12–15
Reverse hyperextension	1 (body weight only)	25–50
Cable crossover	Warmup set (light weight)	10–12
	2–3 (increase poundage each set)	12–15
Machine shoulder press	Warmup set (light weight)	10–12
	2–3 (increase poundage each set)	12–15
Incline side lateral raise	Warmup set (light weight)	10–12
	2–3 (increase poundage each set)	12–15
Low seated pulley row	Warmup set (light weight)	10–12
	2–3 (increase poundage each set)	12–15
Concentration curl	Warmup set (light weight)	10–12
	2–3 (increase poundage each set)	12–15
Machine dip	Warmup set (light weight)	10–12
	2–3 (increase poundage each set)	12–15
Low-pulley triceps extension	Warmup set (light weight)	10–12
	2–3 (increase poundage each set)	12–15
Decline bench crunch	1	15–25

Aerobics

Follow your shape-training routine with 30–45 minutes of walking, jogging or running, or treadmill exercise. Or instead of including an aerobic workout on one of these days, reserve it for Thursday.

*If your gym or workout facility does not have certain types of machines or equipment, refer to Appendix C for exercise substitutions.

TUESDAY

Emphasis:	Fat burning

Aerobics

45 minutes of walking, jogging or running, or treadmill exercise.

WEDNESDAY/SATURDAY

Emphasis:	Midsection specialization

Routine

Exercise	Sets	Repetitions
Decline bench crunch	1–2	15–25
Side crunch	1–2	15–25
Knee-up	1–2	15–25
Dumbbell side bend	1–2	15–25

Aerobics

Follow your midsection specialization routine with 30–45 minutes of walking, jogging or running, or treadmill exercise.

THURSDAY/SUNDAY

Rest

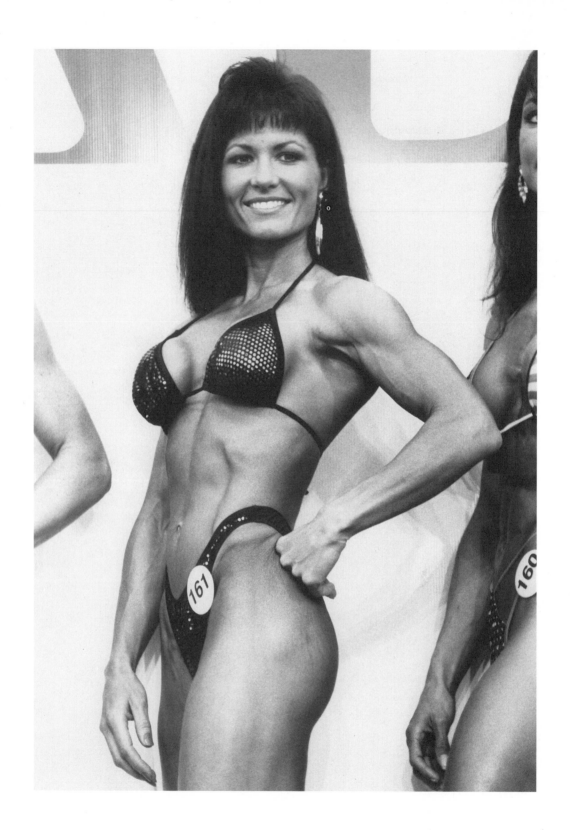

The I-Frame: Adding Curves in All the Right Places

A lot of people are slender and proud of it! And they should be, especially when you consider that so many women are significantly overweight. Still, many thin women want to change their shape by adding curves to their figures. Not only does this improve appearance, it can also have positive benefits on health, as well as improve athletic performance if you play a sport.

Since adding curves means gaining some extra weight, you have to make sure those new pounds are the "right" kind—lean, attractive muscle, not unsightly body fat. The trick is to follow the right kind of exercise program, combined with a weight-gaining diet that's safe and effective. Our diet guidelines for I-frames are outlined in Chapter 13. Those guidelines include information on how many calories you need to put on weight healthfully and which foods are least likely to convert to body fat.

With shape training, you can add curves in all the right places.

How Do I Know Whether I'm Underweight?

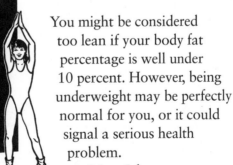

You might be considered too lean if your body fat percentage is well under 10 percent. However, being underweight may be perfectly normal for you, or it could signal a serious health problem.

Most I-frames are generally small-boned, often with a smaller allocation of muscle cells. As an I-frame, you probably have a fast metabolism, too, making it even harder to put on weight and muscle size.

Why Are Some Women Underweight?

Generally, there are several reasons why some people are underweight. The major reasons are heredity, participation in sports, failure to eat enough, and medical problems.

Heredity
You may be destined by heredity to have a very lean figure. It's pretty easy to figure out for yourself whether your frame is genetically rooted. Just ask yourself, Am I built like either of my parents? Are any of my siblings lean? Have I always been slender, even as a kid? If you answered yes to those questions, there's most likely a genetic component to your slenderness.

When genes play a part, you can take heart that there's probably nothing abnormal or unhealthy about your frame. And with the shape-training program outlined in this chapter, you can exercise your body into a more appealing silhouette.

Sports Participation
A lot of women athletes have less than 10 percent body fat. Competitive female runners, for example, may have as little as 5 or 6 percent body fat, according to some studies. A low percentage of body fat or a low weight may be perfectly normal for some women athletes—and desirable because both conditions enhance sports performance. As long as you don't consciously restrict calories while training for a sport, having a naturally lean figure is probably healthy.

Undernutrition
On the other hand, some women are excessively lean because they don't eat enough. Social pressures, such as the strong desire to look like slim fashion models, can lead to undernutrition. An extreme form of undernutrition is *anorexia nervosa,* a life-threatening eating disorder in which the sufferer starves herself to get thin. Symptoms of anorexia include a weight loss of at least 15 percent of original body weight, an abnormal fear of gaining weight, and a distorted body image in which the sufferer thinks she is fat, though in reality she is quite emaciated.

Exercising excessively is another symptom, seen in about 25 percent of anorexic women. Interestingly, therapists now warn anorexic women against doing aerobic exercise because it burns so many calories and draws on fat stores. Instead, they're recommending weight training because it helps distribute weight in a healthful, attractive manner. (If you have any of the symptoms of anorexia nervosa or any type of disordered eating pattern, seek help from a therapist or your physician.)

Another health issue related to undernutrition is *amenorrhea,* the loss of menstrual periods.

Amenorrhea was once associated entirely with leanness and excessive exercise. Having low stores of body fat and exercising a lot appeared to make a woman stop menstruating. But in 1987 a study turned that theory on its ear, finding that many very thin athletes have regular periods. In other words, having a low percentage of body fat and being very active aren't the whole story.

Nutritionists and medical experts now know that amenorrhea has a nutritional component, too. The combination of restricting calories and overexercising depletes body fat stores to unhealthy levels. This depletion leads to an estrogen deficiency, similar to menopause, and your periods cease. There are some side effects to amenorrhea, including premature osteoporosis, heart disease, and inability to become pregnant.

Restarting your periods involves increasing your food intake, getting adequate protein (about half a gram per pound of body weight), and cutting back on exercise. At least 20 percent of your calories should come from fat. You should eat plenty of foods high in iron and calcium. If you have amenorrhea, consult a registered dietitian or physician for professional help.

Medical Problems

You've heard the expression "You can never be too thin, or too rich." Wealth aside, you can most certainly be too thin. In addition to anorexia nervosa and amenorrhea, there are other health-threatening medical conditions related to thinness and weight loss. Examples include hyperthyroidism, in which the metabolism is elevated abnormally; gastrointestinal disorders, in which nutrients are not absorbed properly; and diabetes, which sometimes causes weight loss. If you become thin suddenly and without explanation, seek medical attention immediately.

How Can I Gain Weight in a Healthy Manner?

Gaining the right kind of weight (lean muscle, not fat), in the right places, is mostly a matter of the proper nutrition and a good exercise program. Exercise develops body-shaping muscle where you want it, while good nutrition supplies the calories and nutrients required for building that muscle. Combine the nutrition suggestions for I-frames in Chapter 13 with the exercise routine and recommendations in this chapter, and you'll be on your way to an attractive, healthy new shape in no time at all. In addition to exercise and nutrition, here are a few additional tips to help you:

• *Get adequate rest and sleep.* Without enough shut-eye (eight hours a night is standard for most people), you're using up more calories than you should. This can keep you from gaining weight.

- *Don't smoke.* Smoking accelerates your metabolic rate by as much as 10 percent a day. If you smoke, this habit may be one reason why you've had trouble gaining weight. Stop smoking to curtail your daily energy output.

- *Moderate your use of coffee and other caffeine-containing products.* Caffeine increases your metabolism and keeps it elevated for several hours. Cut back on caffeine to keep your metabolism running in the right gear.

Shape-Training Principles for I-Frames

Several key exercise principles will help you develop lean, body-shaping muscle. These involve the intensity of the exercise, the number of repetitions, the length of time you rest between sets, and the frequency with which you work out. Stick to these principles, and you'll achieve your goal of a curvier figure.

Intensity

To put some extra dimension in your figure, you need to lift heavy poundages, particularly on your last one or two exercise sets. "Heavy" is a relative description; what feels heavy to you might feel light to someone else. The most accurate way to tell what is heavy for you is to identify your *one-rep maximum (1RM)* for each exercise in your shape-training routine. Your 1RM is the most weight you can lift for one repetition. Approximately 80 to 90 percent of your 1RM would be considered a heavy lift.

As an illustration, suppose the most you can lift for one rep on an arm curl exercise is 25 pounds. Eighty percent of that would be about 20 pounds. That's the amount of weight you'd lift on your last set or two.

You'd start your exercise set with a light warmup weight— enough to let you easily do 12 repetitions. Your second set would be a medium poundage—say, about 60 percent of your 1RM, or 15 pounds. Then you'd do your heavy sets at 80 to 90 percent of your 1RM (20 pounds or more).

Here's another way to tell what's heavy: If you can do no more than six or seven repetitions with a given weight, you're working at a heavy intensity.

For your muscles to respond, you have to challenge them to do more. Using the curl as an example again, let's say all you can lift for a while is 20 pounds. A few workouts later, though, that same 20 pounds feels light. Your muscles have adapted to that stress. You now have to challenge them with more weight to keep them in the development mode. That means it's time to add 5 or 10 pounds. From workout to workout, continually strive to stress your muscles progressively beyond what they're used to.

Low Repetitions

In addition to exercising with heavy poundages, you'll employ low repetitions in each set. For enlarging the individual fibers in muscles, the recommendation is 6 to 10 repetitions per set with heavy poundages.

Longer Rest Periods

Rest periods between sets do make a difference, depending on your body type and fitness goals. Women trying to burn body fat, do best with shorter rest periods, since these have a greater calorie-burning effect. But burning up calories isn't your goal. I-frames tend to have fast metabolisms anyway and can use up plenty of calories without even trying. So don't rush through your workout. In your routine, rest one to two minutes between sets. This is considered a long rest break. Try to keep those rest periods as even as possible. Resting one minute here, three minutes there, and so forth could make you lose your concentration.

Exercise Frequency

For results, you should exercise your muscles two to three times a week. The more often you train and challenge your muscles, the faster they will develop. As an I-frame, you'll do best by working your muscles three times a week, with a day or two of rest in between. That's enough time for your muscles to recuperate. During recuperation, your body starts making new muscle.

Shape-Training Exercises for I-Frames

The exercises in your routine are *compound exercises,* meaning that each exercise works several muscles at the same time. Compound exercises are good building exercises. With the exception of abdominal crunches, these exercises use barbells. Barbells stimulate more muscle fibers than other pieces of equipment do and are therefore excellent for developing the shape you seek.

Barbell Squat

Targets: Entire lower body

Be sure to review the guidelines for the squat covered in Chapter 6. To begin, remove the bar from the squat rack and place it behind your neck. Center it on your back. An inch or two off-center can throw your balance way off and be unsafe. Take a step backward from the rack.

Stand with your feet about shoulders' width apart. Keeping your head up, bend your knees and slowly descend. Your back should stay in an erect position. Lower your body until your thighs are slightly below parallel to the floor. Next,

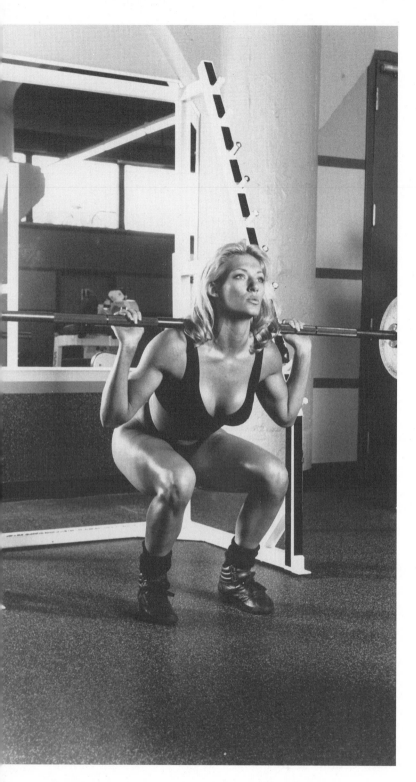

slowly return to the starting position. As you do so, concentrate on using the strength of your thighs and hips to press back up. Upon reaching the top of the exercise (the starting position), squeeze your gluteal (hip) muscles tightly together.

With each repetition, the bar should follow a straight path down to the floor and back up again.

Dead Lift
Targets: Lower body and back

The dead lift is another multimuscle developer—one that works the lower body as well as the back. As with the squat, we recommend that you begin with a light warmup set, using an unloaded bar.

Start with the barbell on the floor. Take a shoulders' width stance and stand so that your lower legs are touching the bar. Grasp the bar with an *alternate grip*—that is, one hand curled under the bar, the other curled over the bar.

Next, bend over the bar, keeping your back flat, knees bent, and head up. Without bending your arms, lift the bar up from the floor until your body is perfectly upright. Lower the bar and repeat the exercise. Concentrate on using the strength of your legs and hips throughout the exercise.

Barbell squat

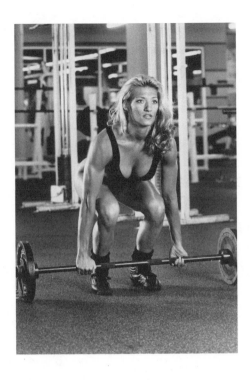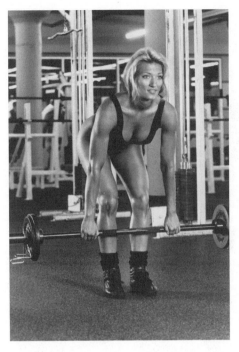

Dead lift

Bent-Over Barbell Row
Targets: Upper back and arms

Perform bent-over barbell rows in front of a mirror to make sure you're positioned correctly. Begin with the barbell on the floor. Bend over so that your back is parallel to the floor, but with a slight arch. Your knees should be bent slightly. Grasp the bar with an overhand grip that's a little wider than shoulders' width. Lift and pull the barbell into your chest. In this position, squeeze the muscles of your upper back. Lower the bar slowly to the starting position. Repeat for the suggested number of repetitions.

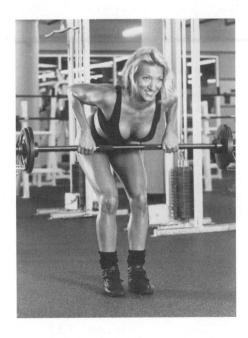

Bent-over barbell row

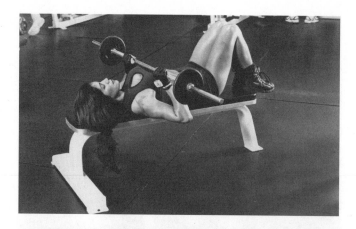

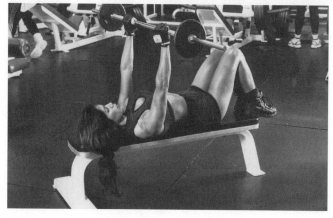

Barbell bench press

Barbell Bench Press
Targets: Pectoral (chest) muscles

Not only does the bench press build the chest, it also develops your shoulders and triceps. Women new to weight training often shy away from the bench press because it seems too macho. That attitude can roadblock your shape-training progress. The bench press is one exercise that quickly and effectively builds attractive—and sexy—upper-body shape.

Now, if you're intimidated by the idea of strength and are afraid to surpass the men in the gym by getting too strong on the bench press, don't worry. You won't beat them on this exercise, because women are 30 to 40 percent weaker in their upper bodies than men are. Women have a much narrower shoulder girth and carry less muscle on the torso than men do—two conditions that greatly limit the amount of upper-body strength you can achieve. Try to explore your own potential for strength without fear. After all, strength is a natural outcome of shape training.

To perform this exercise, lie back on a flat exercise bench and take a grip slightly wider than your shoulders. Using a wide grip distributes the emphasis of the exercise over more muscles.

Lift the bar off the rack to an overhead position. As you progress to heavier weights, a spotter (someone who knows the exercise well enough to coach you) should do this for you. If you don't have a spotter, make sure you use a bench with safety racks that will catch the bar should you fail to complete the lift.

In a slow, controlled motion, lower the bar to your chest to a point about midway between your breasts and shoulder line. Now slowly press back up to a straight-arm position with your elbows locked.

When performing the bench press, concentrate on ultrastrict form. Don't let the bar bounce off your chest during the lowering phase. Bouncing is a bad habit that could injure your chest and rib cage. Nor should you arch your back during the exercise. This action subjects the spine to undue pressure that could lead to injury. To prevent your back from arching, keep your feet flat on the floor and your back pressed close to the bench.

Barbell Shoulder Press
Targets: Shoulders

One of the best exercises for widening the shoulder line is the barbell shoulder press. The shoulder is a three-headed muscle, and this exercise works all three heads, plus the trapezius muscle of the upper back.

We recommend placing the barbell on a rack before beginning the exercise. This saves the energy required to bring it up from the floor. Sit in front of the loaded rack and place your hands on the bar slightly farther apart than shoulders' width. Remove the bar from the rack, and slowly press it upward, locking your elbows at the top. Return to the starting position and continue the exercise for the suggested number of repetitions. After completing the exercise, return the bar to the rack.

Barbell shoulder press

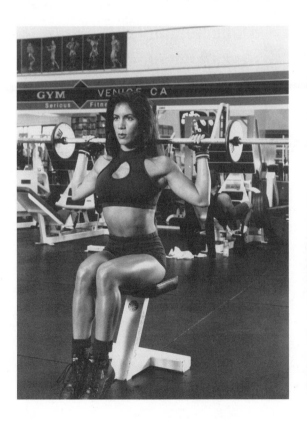
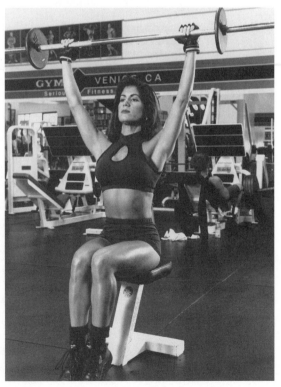

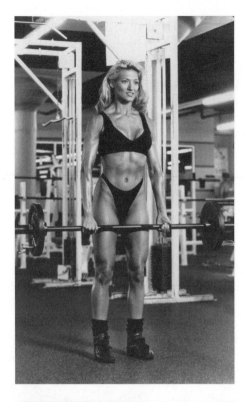

Barbell Curl
Targets: Biceps of arms

To begin, hold the bar so that your grip is slightly wider than shoulders' width. Keep your elbows close to your body. Flex at the elbows, curling the bar upward until it is just under your chin. Slowly return the bar to the starting position. Continue curling for the suggested number of repetitions.

Close-Grip Bench Press
Targets: Triceps (back of upper arms)

The close-grip bench press is to the triceps (the large three-headed muscle at the back of the upper arms) what the barbell curl is to the biceps: a great arm shaper.

We suggest using a *cambered bar*—it's wavy, as opposed to straight—because it's easier to grip during the exercise.

To begin, lie on your back on a flat bench. Have someone hand you the bar, and take a narrow grip in which your hands are about two or three inches apart. Your palms should face toward your feet. Keep your elbows close to your body, then lower the bar to your chest. Press the bar upward and lock your elbows. Slowly lower the bar to your chest. Repeat the exercise.

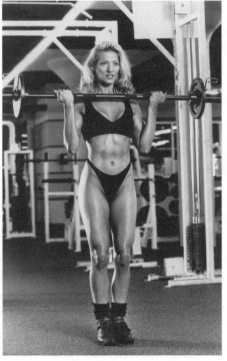

Barbell curl

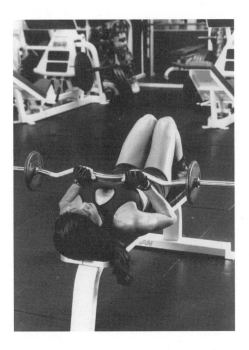
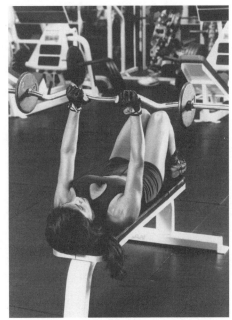

Close-grip bench press

Abdominal Crunch with Weight
Targets: Abdominal muscles

Many women have weak abdominals and lower backs—two muscle groups that are important when performing the squat and dead lift. Your routine includes abdominal crunches because they strengthen these muscles and tone the ab muscles. In this version, you'll use weights for extra firming action.

Lie on your back on the floor with your lower legs draped over a bench. Hold a weight plate in front of your chest. Using the strength of your abdominal muscles, lift your upper torso off the floor toward your thighs. This movement should

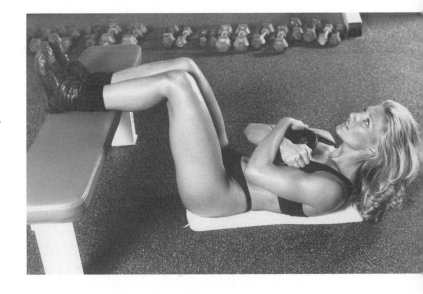

Abdominal crunch with weight

be very short. Don't attempt to actually touch your thighs, as this can overstress your lower back. Keep constant tension on your abdominal muscles throughout the exercise.

How Can I Get Extra-Rapid Results?

It's only natural to want to achieve your desired shape fast. Some recently conducted research sheds light on how you might do this. Researchers at the University of Jyvaskyla in Finland took a group of 10 well-trained women and put them through a three-week weight-training program in which they worked out once a day. Following the first three-week experimentation period, the women trained for another three weeks using the same routine, except this time it was split into two daily sessions. In comparing the results from the two three-week periods, the researchers found that training twice a day, in smaller units, produced significant gains in strength and greater enlargement of muscle fibers.

Though time-consuming, twice-a-day training could get you in shape faster. Plus, it could help you break some plateaus after you've been working out for a while.

To try twice-a-day training, split the following routine into two fairly equal halves. For example, do squats, dead lifts, and bent-over barbell rows in the morning, and the rest of the exercises in the afternoon or evening. You'd still be working out three days a week.

The advantage of doing this is that when you train with just a few exercises, you can really work those body parts hard and long, with even more sets. After working out once a day for at least two months, try this system for three weeks, then return to your regular once-a-day training schedule.

Should Aerobic Exercise Be Part of My Workout?

Include aerobics in your weekly shape-training routine for one important reason: to keep your cardiovascular system in peak condition. However, you don't need to do the kind of high-intensity aerobics that's usually reserved for fat burning. Since you have so little body fat on your frame, there's no need to try to burn any. That could only make you excessively lean. Instead, we suggest some brisk walking two or three times a week for 20 to 30 minutes. Or try swimming, since it tends to conserve body weight.

Shape-Training Routine: I-Frames

MONDAY/WEDNESDAY/FRIDAY

Emphasis:	Total body development and shaping
Warmup:	5–10 minutes of relaxed walking
Exercise style:	Heavy weights and low repetitions (6–10)

Routine

Exercise*	Sets	Repetitions
Barbell squat	Set 1: Warmup set with unloaded bar	12–15
	Set 2: Medium poundage	10–12
	Set 3: Heavy poundage	6–10
	Set 4: Heavy poundage	6–8
Dead lift	Set 1: Warmup set with unloaded bar	12–15
	Set 2: Medium poundage	10–12
	Set 3: Heavy poundage	6–10
Bent-over barbell row	Set 1: Warmup set with unloaded bar	12–15
	Set 2: Medium poundage	10–12
	Set 3: Heavy poundage	6–10
Barbell bench press	Set 1: Warmup set with unloaded bar	12–15
	Set 2: Medium poundage	10–12
	Set 3: Heavy poundage	6–10
	Set 4: Heavy poundage	6–8
Barbell shoulder press	Set 1: Warmup set with unloaded bar	12–15
	Set 2: Medium poundage	10–12
	Set 3: Heavy poundage	6–10
Barbell curl	Set 1: Warmup set with unloaded bar	12–15
	Set 2: Medium poundage	10–12
	Set 3: Heavy poundage	6–10
Close-grip bench press	Set 1: Warmup set with unloaded bar	12–15
	Set 2: Medium poundage	10–12
	Set 3: Heavy poundage	6–10
Abdominal crunch with weight	1	Start with 10 or 12; over time, try to work up to 50

TUESDAY/THURSDAY/SATURDAY

Emphasis:	Cardiovascular fitness

Do 20–30 minutes of moderate to fast-paced walking or swimming to keep your cardiovascular system in good condition.

SUNDAY

Rest

---

*If your gym or workout facility does not have certain types of machines or equipment, refer to Appendix C for exercise substitutions.

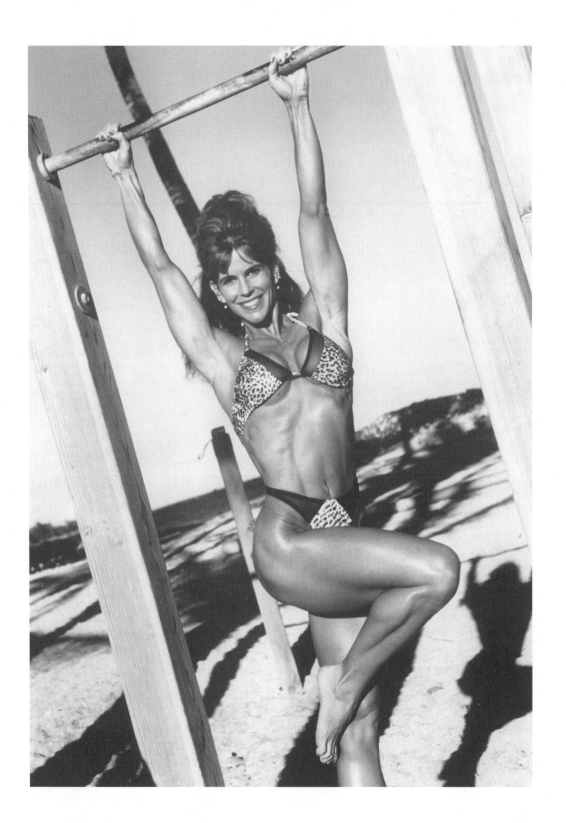

The O-Frame: Paring Off Pounds

If you have an O-frame, burning fat is your foremost concern, since you have a higher percentage of body fat to lean muscle and a slow metabolism. Often, though, fighting fat is like trying to roller-skate uphill—practically impossible! And there's certainly no shortage of diets to help with the fight. Many overweight people will try just about any diet that comes around the bend, regardless of how unhealthy or unsafe it might be. Yet very few people are willing to give exercise a fair shake.

Despite the umpteen diets around, the best counsel is still this: Burn more calories than you eat, and you'll deplete your fat stores and slowly strip them away. The easiest way to use up more calories is to get more active. Physical activity is an essential part of fat loss,

particularly since it increases your metabolism and makes your body more efficient at burning fat. Without exercise, you're more likely to put the lost pounds right back on.

Using specific shape-training techniques, you can get firm—fast. (Model: Debbie Kaniko)

Shape Training Geared for Fat Loss

You have three shape-training options for burning fat. Routine 1 is designed for people who are new to weight training. Its goal is to develop firm, calorie-burning muscle. You need more muscle on your body to increase your metabolism and burn fat. Routine 1 also tones and tightens all key muscle groups. You should supplement this routine with aerobics three to five times a week. Guidelines for increasing the frequency and duration of your aerobics are given later in this chapter.

Routine 2 is a special kind of workout known as *circuit training,* an aerobic-type program designed for muscle toning and fat burning. Each "circuit" is a series of exercises, performed in nonstop sequence. You rest for a minute or two after each circuit, then repeat the circuit one or two more times. This routine is ideal if you're on a tight time schedule but want to lose body fat relatively quickly. Since this routine is aerobic all by itself, you need to do regular aerobics only two or three times a week.

Once you've used Routines 1 or 2 for six to eight weeks, try Routine 3, a split routine known as a four-day-on/one-day-off system. You work your body as follows:

- Day 1—Legs, abdominals
- Day 2—Back, abdominals, aerobics
- Day 3—Chest, shoulders, abdominals
- Day 4—Arms, abdominals, aerobics
- Day 5—Aerobics or Rest
- Day 6—Begin repeating the cycle

Routine 3 is an advanced routine designed to increase your weekly calorie expenditure for fat burning and further define, sculpt, and shape your muscles. You do abdominal exercises four days a week, since abs often need extra work if you're an O-frame. Also, you perform slightly higher repetitions (12 to 15) on all upper-body exercises and even more on leg and abdominal exercises (15 to 25), plus extra sets. Higher repetitions and additional sets provide an aerobic effect to stimulate fat burning. Use weights heavy enough to make you work hard, but light enough to do the desired number of sets and repetitions. Routine 3 includes aerobics to increase fat burning.

When you are performing Routines 1 and 3, it's important that you keep your rest between sets to a minimum.

Exercise Safety Guidelines for O-Frames

Many O-frames with a lot of weight to lose have not exercised much in the past and therefore should ease into an exercise program, increasing their effort level very gradually. With that in mind, here's some advice for nonexercisers who want to get more active:

- If you're "formerly inactive"— that is, you've never done much exercise before—increase your activity level in everyday activities before engaging in a formal exercise routine. Park farther away while shopping so you can walk to the store, or choose the stairs over the elevator, for example.

- After a few weeks of increasing daily activity, begin your shape-training program. For the first several weeks, use only light to moderate poundages. This will help increase calorie-burning lean muscle. Gradually work up to heavier weights by adding a little weight (two to five pounds) to each exercise week by week.
- Do aerobic exercise at least three days a week for at least 20 to 30 minutes. Work out at a pace at which you can still carry on a conversation. This should put you at roughly 60 to 80 percent of your maximum heart rate—enough to burn between 1,500 and 2,000 calories a week.
- Gradually try to work up to 45 minutes of aerobic exercise four to five times a week.
- Stay consistent in your exercise program.

Best Aerobic Choices for O-Frames

For permanent fat loss, choose aerobic exercises that work the entire body or at least large muscle groups. These expend more calories and build overall fitness. Walking is one of the easiest—and safest—activities for burning calories and tuning up the cardiovascular system. If you opt for walking, walk as long as you can. In a study of obese women who progressively increased their periods of walking over a year's time, no weight loss occurred until walking exceeded 30 minutes. All the weight they lost was pure fat.

Walking may not be the best bet, however, for anyone who is very overweight (a body fat percentage exceeding 35 percent), since these people often have joint problems. If that's the case, try activities such as stationary cycling, rowing, or using cross-country ski machines. These place less stress on the joints.

Swimming is often recommended as an exercise option for very overweight people because it is easy on the joints, too. But as noted earlier, it doesn't measure up as well for fat loss as other forms of aerobic activity.

The best exercise bet for you will be the one you most enjoy. Whatever you choose, get the blessing of your physician before starting any exercise program.

Shape-Training Exercises for O-Frames

The shape-training routines for O-frames are aimed at toning the whole body, boosting metabolism, and encouraging weight loss.

Leg Press
Targets: Thighs and buttocks

Position yourself in the leg press machine so that your feet are about

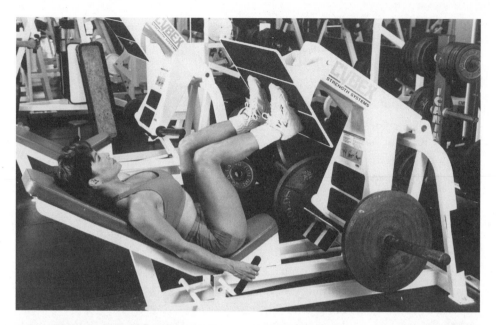

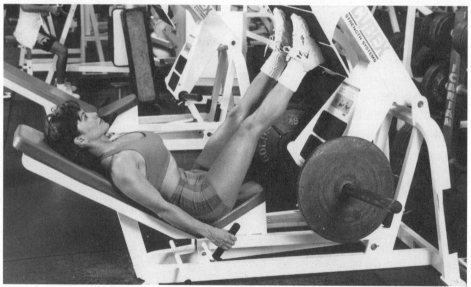

Leg press

a foot apart. Release the safety stops, and lower the platform slowly to bring your knees to your chest. Press forward until your legs are fully extended, locking out your knees at the top. Continue pressing in this manner for the suggested number of repetitions.

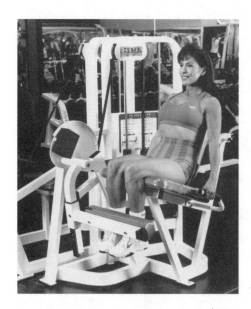

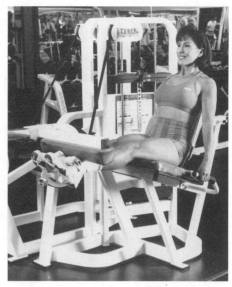

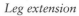
Leg extension

Leg Extension
Targets: Thighs

Sit in the leg extension machine, and hook the insteps of your feet under the padded roller. Curl the roller up in an arc until your legs are parallel to the floor. Lock your knees out, and hold this position for a second or two. Then return slowly to the starting position. Control the movement at all times. Try not to kick the weight up, since this will force momentum to take over, and the exercise will be less effective. Repeat the exercise for the suggested number of repetitions.

Standing Leg Curl
Targets: Hamstrings

Performed on a special machine, the standing leg curl isolates the muscles at the rear of the thigh. Stand in the machine, and place the ankle of one leg under the padded roller. Bring your heel toward your buttocks. Lower slowly to the starting position. Repeat. Complete your set, then work the other leg.

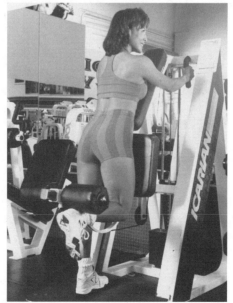

Standing leg curl

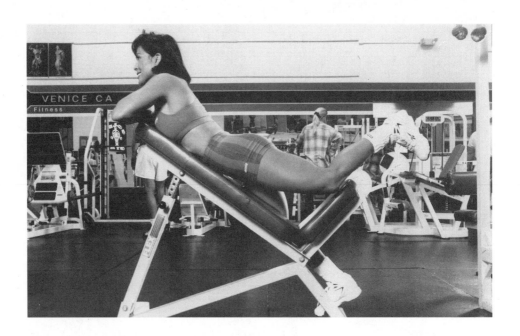

Incline back kick

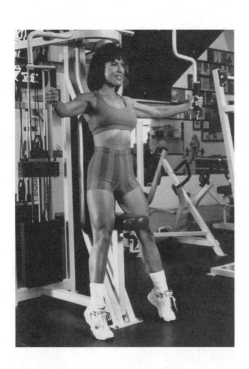
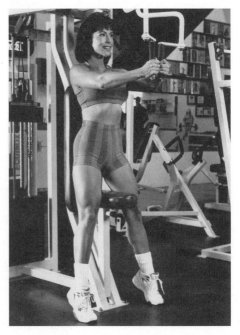

Machine chest fly

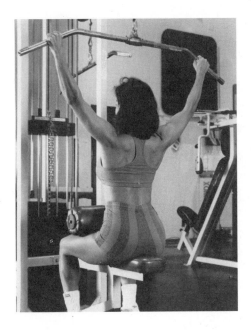

Incline Back Kick
Targets: Buttocks and hamstrings

The incline back kick firms up the rear of the buttocks and the tops of the hamstrings—an area that tends to sag, yet benefits from extra exercise attention. Lie face forward on a full-length incline board, and hold onto the edges of the board for support. With your knee slightly bent, raise your right leg up behind you as far as you can. Squeeze your buttocks as tightly as possible. Perform as many repetitions as you can, up to 25 or 30. Repeat the exercise with the left leg.

Machine Chest Fly
Targets: Pectoral (chest) muscles

Sit in the fly machine and place the inner side of your forearms against each pad. Press the pads forward until they meet in front of your chest, squeezing your pectoral muscles hard. Continue pressing the pads inward and outward to complete your exercise set.

Wide-Grip Pulldown
Targets: Upper back

Perform the wide-grip pulldown on a cable machine using a long bar. Sit facing the machine, and take an overhand grip on the bar. Your grip should be slightly wider than shoulders' width. Pull the bar down behind your neck as far as you can. In this position, arch your back slightly to emphasize your upper-back muscles. Slowly return the bar to the starting position. Repeat the exercise for the suggested number of repetitions.

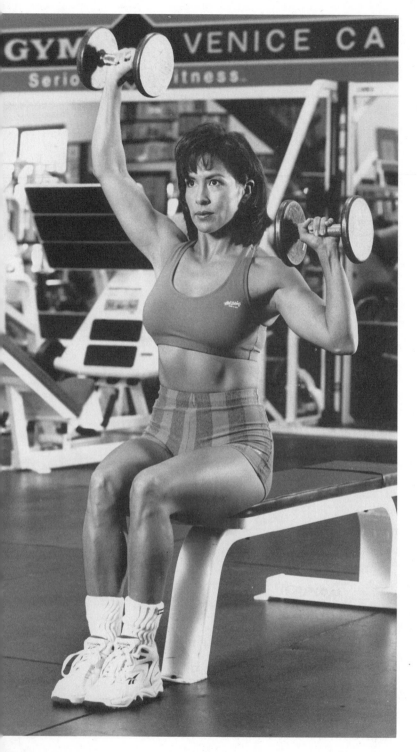

Seated Alternating Dumbbell Press
Targets: Shoulders

Sit on an exercise bench, and take a dumbbell in each hand. Hold them at shoulder level, palms facing forward. Press the right dumbbell upward to an overhead position. As you begin to lower the right dumbbell, start pressing the left dumbbell upward to an overhead position. When the right dumbbell is at the starting position, the left one should be in the overhead position. Continue alternating in this manner for the suggested number of repetitions.

Seated Alternating Dumbbell Curl
Targets: Biceps of arms

Sit on an exercise bench, holding a dumbbell in each hand. With your upper arms pressed close to your sides, curl the right dumbbell up, palms facing upward, until it reaches shoulder level. As you begin to lower the right dumbbell, start curling the left dumbbell up in the same manner. When the right dumbbell is at the starting position, the left one should be at shoulder level. Continue alternating in this manner for the suggested number of repetitions.

Seated alternating dumbbell press

Single-Arm Pulley Pressdown
Targets: Triceps (back of upper arm)

Hold a cable handle in your right
hand, holding your upper arm
against the side of your torso. Press
your lower right arm down in an arc
until it is fully straightened. Slowly
return to the starting position, and
continue the exercise for the suggested number of repetitions. Repeat
the exercise with the left arm.

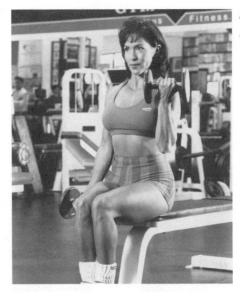

*Seated alternating
dumbbell curl*

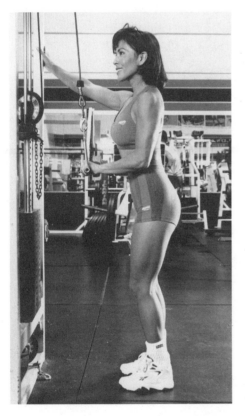

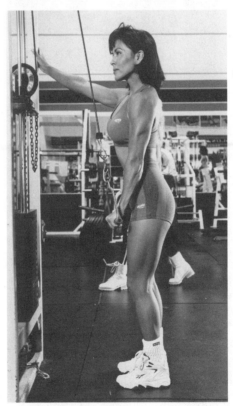

Single-arm pulley pressdown

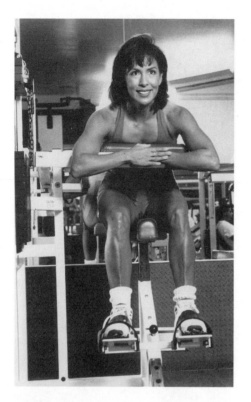

Abdominal machine

Abdominal Machine
Targets: Abdominal muscles

There are many different makes and models of abdominal machines. Most simulate the action of the crunch exercise and let you easily add weight to the exercise to better stimulate the abdominal muscles.

To begin, properly position yourself in the machine according to its design. Next, bring your torso toward your knees, using the strength of your abdominal muscles, not your back. Squeeze your abs together tightly in the contracted position. Continue the exercise for as many repetitions as you can.

Seated Calf Raise
Targets: Calves

The seated calf raise tones the lower leg. Sit in the machine and adjust the padded bar so that it fits snugly across your knees. Raise your heels as high as you can, then lower them as deeply as you can for a good stretch. Continue raising and lowering in this manner for as many reps as you can.

The muscles of the calves respond best to high repetitions.

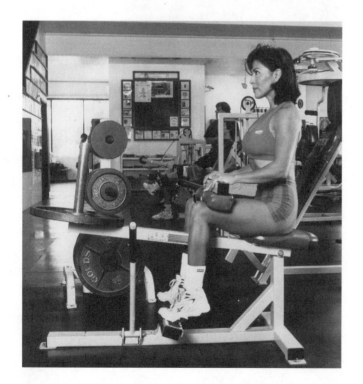

Seated calf raise

Shape-Training Routine: O-Frames, Routine 1

MONDAY/WEDNESDAY/FRIDAY

Emphasis:	Building metabolism, overall toning, and losing body fat
Warmup:	5–10 minutes of relaxed walking
Exercise style:	Moderate to heavy poundages with medium reps (10–12) to low reps (6–10)

Routine

Exercise*	Sets	Repetitions
Leg press	Set 1: Warmup (light weight)	10–12
	Set 2: Moderate weight	10–12
	Set 3: Heavy weight	6–10
Leg extension	Set 1: Warmup (light weight)	10–12
	Set 2: Moderate to heavy weight	8–10
	Set 3: Heavy weight	6–8
Standing leg curl	Set 1: Warmup (light weight)	10–12
	Set 2: Moderate to heavy weight	8–10
	Set 3: Heavy weight	6–8
Incline back kick	1	Up to 30
Machine chest fly	Set 1: Warmup (light weight)	15
	Set 2: Moderate weight	10–12
	Set 3: Heavy weight	6–10
Wide-grip pulldown	Set 1: Warmup (light weight)	15
	Set 2: Moderate weight	10–12
	Set 3: Heavy weight	6–10
Seated alternating dumbbell press	Set 1: Warmup (light weight)	15 on each arm
	Set 2: Moderate weight	10–12 on each arm
	Set 3: Heavy weight	6–10 on each arm
Seated alternating dumbbell curl	Set 1: Warmup (light weight)	15 on each arm
	Set 2: Moderate weight	10–12 on each arm
	Set 3: Heavy weight	6–10 on each arm
Single-arm pulley pressdown	Set 1: Warmup (light weight)	15 on each arm
	Set 2: Moderate weight	10–12 on each arm
	Set 3: Heavy weight	6–10 on each arm
Abdominal machine	1 (moderate weight)	Up to 25
Seated calf raise	1 (moderate weight)	25–50

Aerobics

Follow each workout with 20–30 minutes of aerobic exercise. Choices include brisk walking, swimming, stationary cycling, stair climbing, or cross-country skiing on a machine.

TUESDAY/THURSDAY/SATURDAY
Aerobics

As you become more aerobically fit, perform aerobic exercise on additional days during the week. Try to gradually work up to four or more aerobic sessions a week, 30 to 45 minutes each time.

SUNDAY

Rest

---

*If your gym or workout facility does not have certain types of machines or equipment, refer to Appendix C for exercise substitutions.

Shape-Training Routine: O-Frames, Routine 2 (Circuit Training)

MONDAY/WEDNESDAY/FRIDAY

Emphasis:	Building metabolism, overall toning, and losing body fat
Warmup:	5–10 minutes of relaxed walking
Exercise style:	Moderate poundages with medium reps (10–12) on most exercises

Routine

Exercise*	Sets**	Repetitions**
Leg press	1	10–12
Leg extension	1	10–12
Standing leg curl	1	10–12
Incline back kick	1	Up to 30
Machine chest fly	1	10–12
Wide-grip pulldown	1	10–12
Seated alternating dumbbell press	1	10–12
Seated alternating dumbbell curl	1	10–12
Single-arm pulley pressdown	1	10–12
Abdominal machine	1	Up to 25
Seated calf raise	1	25–50

TUESDAY/SATURDAY

Aerobics

Perform aerobics 30 to 45 minutes each session. Choices include brisk walking, swimming, stationary cycling, stair climbing, or cross-country skiing on a machine.

THURSDAY/SUNDAY

Rest

*If your gym or workout facility does not have certain types of machines or equipment, refer to Appendix C for exercise substitutions.

**Repeat the circuit two more times, increasing the poundage while lowering the repetitions (8–10) on each exercise.

Shape-Training Routine: O-Frame, Routine 3
(Advanced Fat-Burning Routine)

4 DAYS ON/1 DAY OFF

Emphasis:	Overall toning and fat loss
Warmup:	5–10 minutes of relaxed walking
Exercise style:	Moderate poundages with high repetitions

DAY 1   LEGS AND ABDOMINALS

Exercise*	Sets**	Repetitions
Leg press	4–5	15–25
Leg extension	4–5	15–25
Standing leg curl	4–5	15–25
Incline back kick	4–5	15–25
Seated calf raise	4–5	15–25
Abdominal machine	2–3	15–25

DAY 2   BACK AND ABDOMINALS

Exercise*	Sets**	Repetitions
Wide-grip pulldown	4–5	12–15
Abdominal machine	2–3	15–25

Aerobics

Perform 30–45 minutes of brisk walking, weighted walking, jogging or running, or Crossrobics.

DAY 3   CHEST, SHOULDERS, AND ABDOMINALS

Exercise*	Sets**	Repetitions
Machine chest fly	4–5	12–15
Seated alternating dumbbell press	4–5	12–15
Abdominal machine	2–3	15–25

DAY 4   ARMS AND ABDOMINALS

Exercise*	Sets**	Repetitions
Seated alternating dumbbell curl	4–5	12–15
Single-arm pulley pressdown	4–5	12–15
Abdominal machine	2–3	15–25

Aerobics

Perform 30–45 minutes of brisk walking, weighted walking, stationary cycling, or Crossrobics.

DAY 5   REST OR AEROBICS

Perform 30–45 minutes of brisk walking, weighted walking, stationary cycling, or Crossrobics.

DAY 6   BEGIN REPEATING CYCLE

---

*If your gym or workout facility does not have certain types of machines or equipment, refer to Appendix C for exercise substitutions.

**The first set should be a warmup set with a light weight.

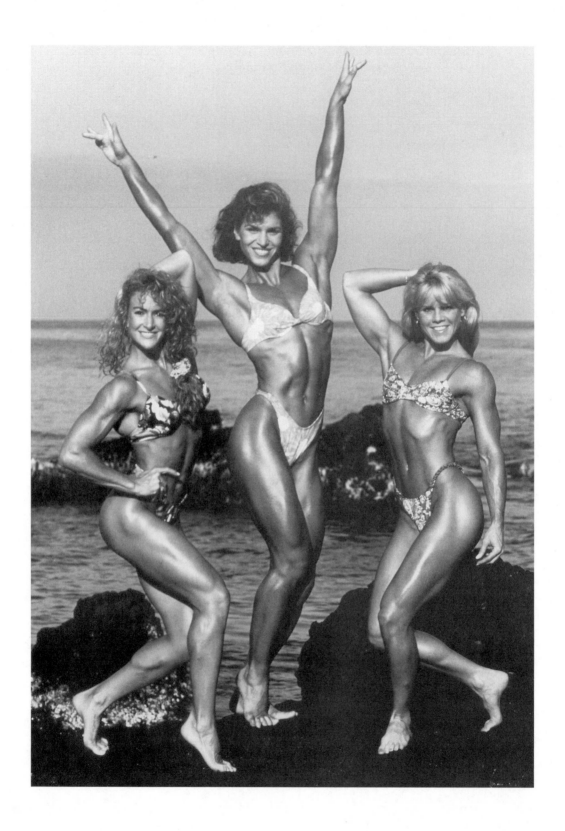

10

The T-Frame: Trimming a Top-Heavy Figure

The T-frame—slender legs and hips, coupled with an amply endowed upper body—has great shape-training potential. All you have to do is tighten upper-body trouble spots and recontour your lower body so that it's a little curvier. Achieving both goals will shift your proportions so that you're less top-loaded. You can do it with the right exercise methods and fat-burning aerobics.

Besides appearance, there are significant reasons to pare down if you're a T with too much on top. As noted in Chapter 3, upper-body fat is a risk factor for hormone-related cancers such as breast cancer, as well as for heart disease. In contrast, having a strong, well-developed upper body enables you to accomplish day-to-day tasks. If you participate in a sport, you have the stamina and power to throw farther, swing harder, hit more powerfully. Upper-body strength even helps if you're a runner; the faster you can move your arms, the faster you can run. A strong upper body protects you against potential athletic injuries, particularly in your shoulders and back. Getting stronger can even alleviate everyday aches and pains, such as lower-back problems, caused by muscular weakness.

Mia Finnegan, Marjo Selin, and Shannon Meteraud use all the right exercise techniques to balance their figures.

Upper-Body Trimming Techniques

To reshape your upper body, you'll use a technique known as *supersets*. Basically, these are combinations of two different exercises for the same muscle, performed one right after the other with no rest in between.

This kind of training, particularly when performed with high reps and moderate weights, increases muscle tone. Supersets also enhance the fat-burning process, since the exercises are to be performed in rapid succession.

Another advantage of supersets is that they're time-efficient. With supersets, you do more work but in less time. That's always a plus for today's on-the-go exercisers.

You'll definitely feel a burn in your muscles when you use supersets. This method of exercising produces a significant amount of waste products, namely lactic acid, in the muscle. The buildup of lactic acid causes the burning feeling and results from a lack of oxygen in the working muscles. The burn subsides during your rest breaks, when oxygen is resupplied to your muscles. The more fit you become, the longer you can exercise before experiencing the burn.

Following are 10 sure-shapers for your upper body, with instructions on how to combine them into supersets.

Incline dumbbell chest press

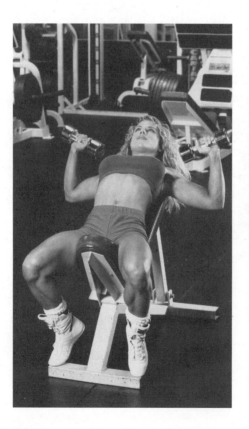
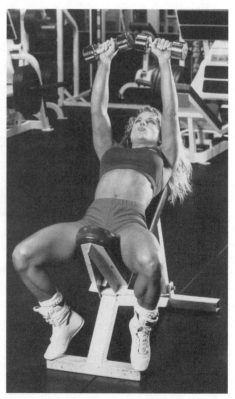

Incline Dumbbell Chest Press/Incline Dumbbell Fly

Targets: Pectoral (chest) muscles

To perform the incline dumbbell chest press, hold two dumbbells and lie on an incline bench situated at a 45-degree angle. Begin with the weights at chest level, palms pointing forward. Press the weights upward, then lower slowly to the starting position. Repeat this exercise for the suggested number of repetitions. After completing your repetitions, immediately begin the incline dumbbell fly exercise.

For the incline dumbbell fly, lie on your back on the incline bench with the two dumbbells held out in front of you in a straight-arm position. Flex your elbows slightly and lower the weights slowly out to the sides of your body. Get a good stretch at bottom (the lowest point you can go with the weights). Then return to the starting position. Repeat this exercise for the suggested number of repetitions. Rest 30 to 45 seconds before repeating the superset.

Incline dumbbell fly

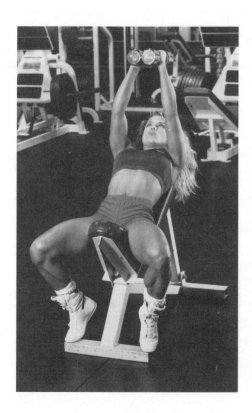
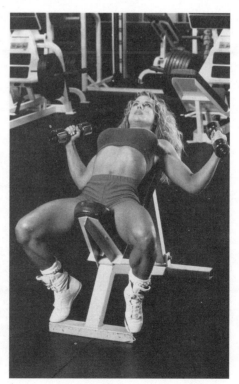

Side lateral raise

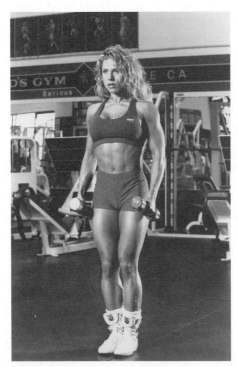
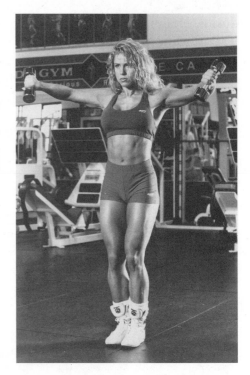

Rear lateral raise

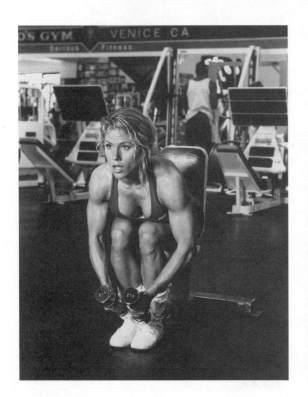
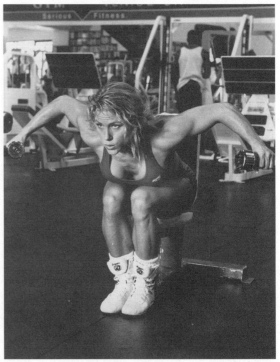

SHAPE TRAINING

Side Lateral Raise/Rear Lateral Raise
Targets: Shoulders

You can perform side lateral raises in a seated or standing position. To begin the exercise, hold a dumbbell in each hand held at your sides. Keeping your elbows slightly bent, raise the dumbbells up at your sides to shoulder level. Lower your arms to your sides. Repeat for the suggested number of repetitions. Upon completing your last rep, immediately begin the rear lateral raise exercise.

Rear lateral raises are best performed in a seated position. Bend forward so that your upper body is touching your knees. Your upper body should be parallel to the floor. Both dumbbells should be in front of your feet on the floor.

To begin, take a dumbbell in each hand and lift them out to the sides of your body as high as you can. Squeeze your rear shoulder muscles at the top of the exercise. Lower to the starting position. Repeat for the suggested number of repetitions. Rest 30 to 45 seconds and repeat the superset.

Dumbbell Rowing/High-Pulley Rowing
Targets: Upper back

To begin the dumbbell rowing exercise, bend over so that your upper body is parallel to the floor. Place one hand on a bench for balance. In the other hand, hold a dumbbell with your arm extended straight down. Flexing your arm, pull the weight directly up to the side of your chest. Squeeze your back muscles at the top of the exercise. Lower the weight to the starting position. Repeat for the suggested number of repetitions. Repeat the exercise with the other arm. After your last rep, immediately begin the next exercise in your superset.

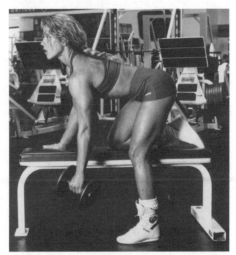

Dumbbell rowing

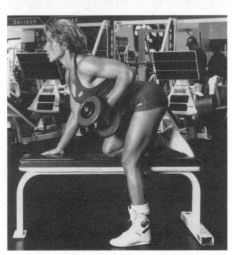

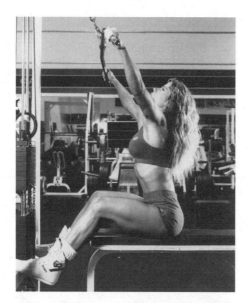

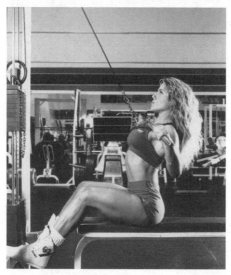

Perform the high-pulley rowing exercise at a cable machine. Sit with your legs extended straight out in front of you. Secure your feet against the machine's foot pad. Hold the cable bar, then pull it directly into your upper chest. Squeeze your back muscles by pulling your shoulder blades together, and hold for a

second or two. Then straighten your arms and return to the starting position. Repeat the exercise for the suggested number of repetitions. Rest 30 to 45 seconds and repeat the superset.

Cable Curl/Inner-Biceps Curl
Targets: Biceps of arms

Cable curls are performed at a cable machine. Attach handles to the left and right high-pulley apparatus, and select a weight with which you can do 12 to 15 repetitions with some intensity of effort. Stand between the two pulley stations, and grip each handle as shown. Begin the exercise with your arms extended out. Now bend your elbows until your hands reach your head. Hold this flexed position for a few seconds. Then return slowly to the starting position. Repeat for the suggested number of repetitions. After your last rep, move on to the inner-biceps curl.

To begin the inner-biceps curl, take a dumbbell in each hand and hold them at your sides with your palms facing in. As you start the exercise, curl your wrists so your palms are facing forward, bend your elbows, and raise the weights out to your sides. Keep your upper arms pressed close to your body. Lower the weights slowly. Repeat the exercise for the suggested number of repetitions. Rest 30 to 45 seconds and repeat the superset.

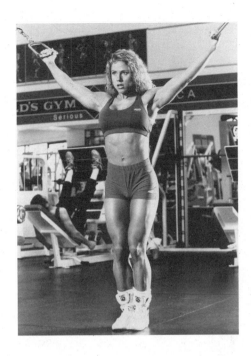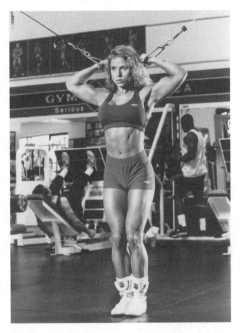

Cable curl

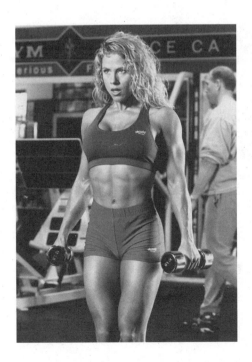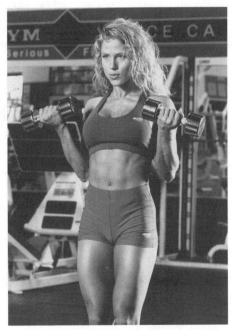

Inner-biceps curl

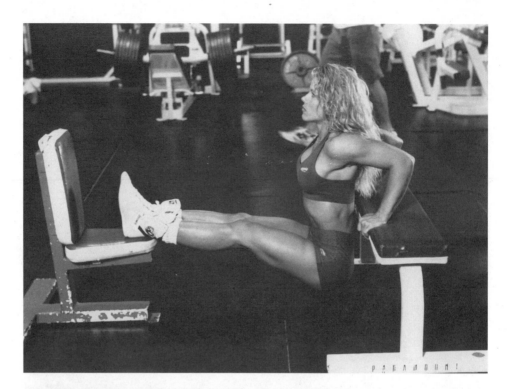

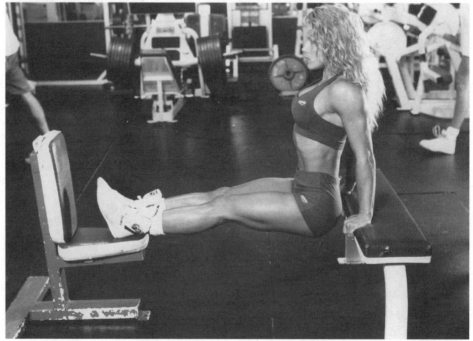

Bench dip

SHAPE TRAINING

Bench Dip/Overhead Triceps Extension
Targets: Triceps (back of upper arm)

For bench dips, place two flat benches parallel to each other, about a leg's length apart. Situate your body between the two benches with your back to one of them. Grasp the edge of the bench behind you, with your forearms and fingers pointing forward. Extend your legs, and place your ankles and feet on the facing bench. Bend your elbows, and slowly lower your hips toward the floor. Push yourself back up, and lock your elbows at the top of the exercise. Lower and repeat for as many repetitions as you can, up to 15. Follow this exercise with overhead triceps extensions.

You can perform the overhead triceps extension exercise in a seated position. Hold one dumbbell with both hands behind your head. Your elbows should be bent and pressed close to the sides of your head. Raise the dumbbell upward to an overhead position. Lock your elbows at the top of the exercise. Lower the dumbbell. Repeat the exercise for the suggested number of repetitions.

Overhead triceps extension

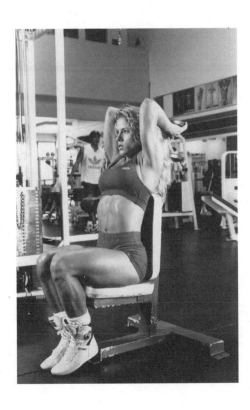
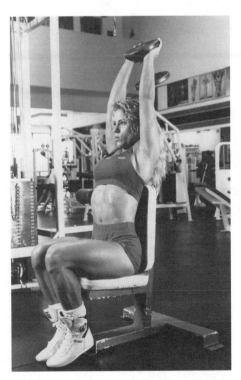

Curve Builders for the Lower Body

As a T-frame, you may not need to trim your thighs and hips, but you do need some curves to balance your proportions. The shape-training routine for your lower body concentrates on achieving that goal. You'll do some proven curve builders with low repetitions and heavier weights—the best rep/poundage combo for adding extra dimensions.

Close-Stance Half Squat
Targets: Outer thighs

To begin the close-stance half squat, place a barbell on your shoulders behind your neck and hold it there with both hands. Stand with your feet just a few inches apart and your toes pointing straight forward. Keeping your back erect and your head up, slowly bend your knees slightly—to a point at which your thighs are at a 45-degree angle to the floor. This is a very slight bend. Try to keep tension on your thighs throughout the exercise. A word of caution: Don't try to descend to a position where your thighs are parallel to the floor; you'd have to bend over too much.

Slowly stand back up and return to the starting point. Repeat the movement. Perform squats with a poundage at which you can handle the suggested number of repetitions.

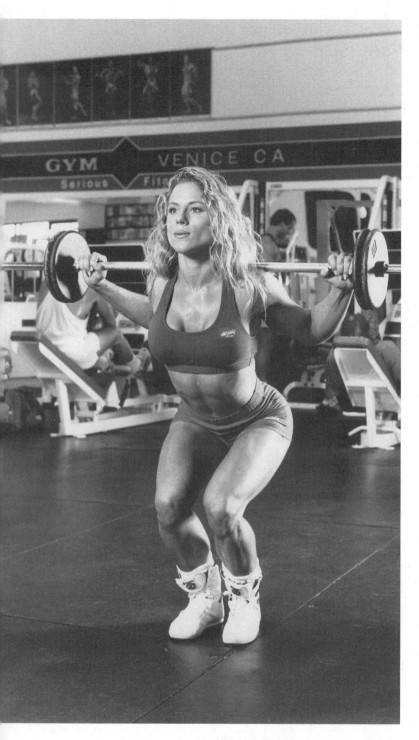

Close-stance half squat

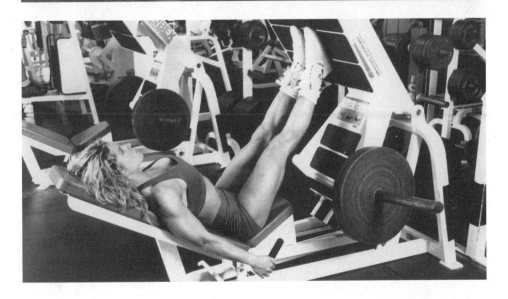

Close-Stance Leg Press
Targets: Outer thighs

Keeping your feet close together puts the emphasis of this leg press exercise on your outer thighs. Position yourself in the machine with your feet placed a few inches apart on the foot pads. Press forward until your legs are straight. Lock your knees. Bend your knees and bring them toward your upper body. Continue pressing in this fashion for the suggested number of repetitions.

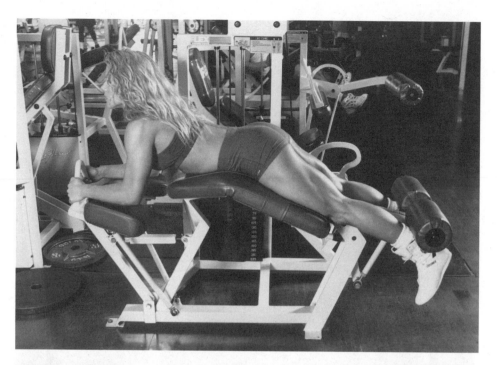

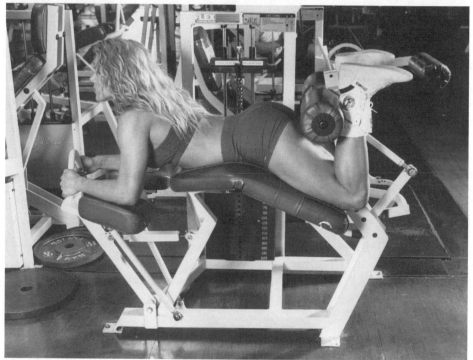

Leg curl

SHAPE TRAINING

Leg Curl
Targets: Hamstrings and buttocks

Leg curls require a special machine. Lying face down on the machine's bench, hook your ankles under the padded rollers. Flex at the knees, bringing your ankles toward your hips in an arc. At the top of the exercise, squeeze your buttocks together. Lower slowly. Repeat for the suggested number of repetitions.

Standing Calf Raise
Targets: Calves

To do the standing calf raise, you need a special machine. Select a fairly light weight for this exercise. Position yourself in the machine so that your shoulders are underneath the pads and the balls of your feet are on the platform. Rise up and down, getting a good stretch in the lower position.

Because the muscle fibers of the calves are tightly compacted, they benefit from high repetitions.

Abdominal Work for T-Frames

Many T-frames need to firm up their abdominal muscles for a better shape. Strong ab muscles also enhance posture. Remember, abdominal exercises won't remove flab, but

Standing calf raise

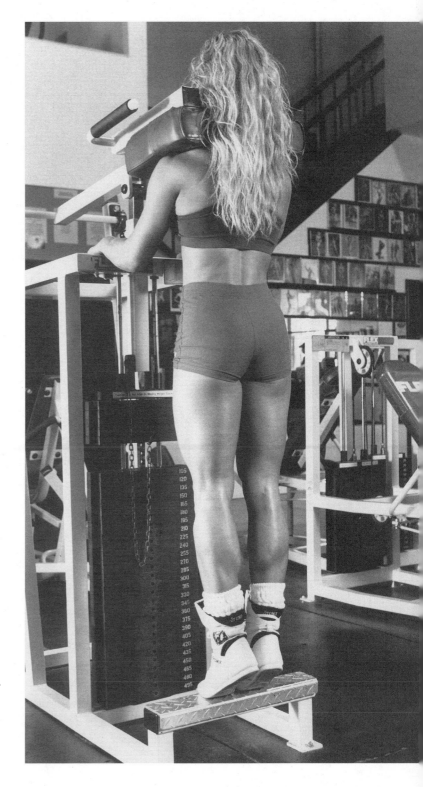

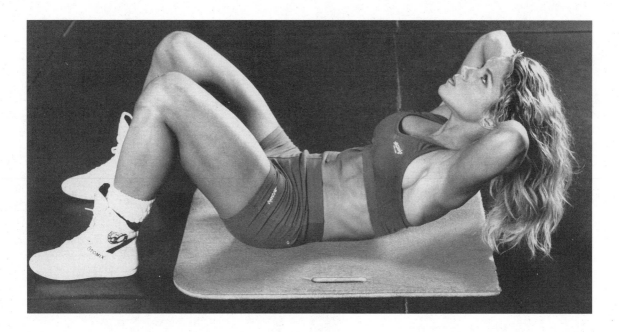

Floor crunch

they will tighten up the muscles underneath. In fact, abs are one of the easiest body spots to shape up. Here are two excellent all-around abdominal exercises to include in your shape-training routine.

Floor Crunch

The floor crunch is a version of the standard crunch that works the entire abdominal wall. The special position of the body places very little pressure on the lower back.

Lie on your back with your legs on the floor and your knees bent. Place your hands behind your head, and keep your elbows pointing outward. Bring your upper body and shoulders off the floor slightly, using the strength of your abdominal muscles. Return to the starting position and repeat.

Like the calf muscles, the abs benefit from high-repetition exercise.

Seated Reverse Crunch

Sit on a chair or a seated workout bench, close to its edge. Grasp the sides of the chair with your hands and lean backward, resting your back on the back of the chair. Bend your knees and bring them toward your chest. Extend them straight out in front. Return to the starting position. Continue the exercise for the suggested number of repetitions.

Concentrate on using the strength of your abdominal muscles

to push through the exercise. Otherwise, you could place too much stress on your lower back.

Accelerating Fat Loss with Aerobics

Fat loss is an issue for many T-frames. If you need to shed body fat, we suggest that you try to fit in four to five aerobic sessions a week for some extra calorie burning. You can do these following your upper-body and lower-body workouts. There's a fat-burning advantage in this as well: By the time you've finished your shape-training workout, you've used up plenty of stored carbohydrate in your muscles. As noted earlier, this forces your body to start burning fat for fuel once you start performing aerobics. By doing aerobics after your shape-training routine, you make the switch to fat metabolism much faster and get leaner as a result.

Good aerobics choices for T-frames are ones that use the large muscles of the body, particularly if you want to burn body fat. Here are some examples:

- Crossrobics
- Stair climbing
- Stationary cycling
- Cross-country ski machine
- Weighted walking
- Rowing machine

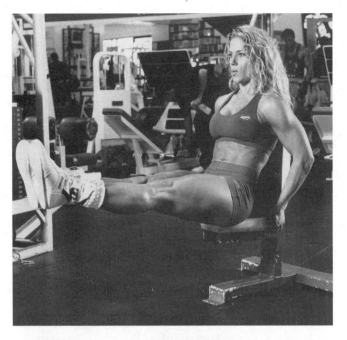

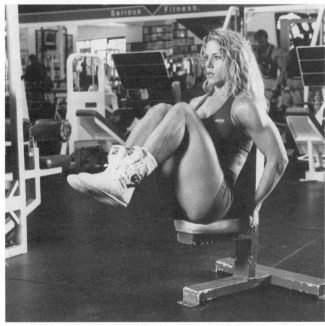

Seated reverse crunch

Shape-Training Routine for T-Frames

Your routine is a four-day split. You concentrate on upper-body toning on Monday and Thursday, lower-body building on Tuesday and Friday. Try to do your aerobics on those four days as well, and include a fifth aerobic workout on Saturday.

Shape-Training Routine: T-Frames

MONDAY/THURSDAY

Emphasis:	Upper-body toning
Warmup:	5–10 minutes of relaxed walking
Exercise style:	Supersets using moderate weights and high repetitions (12–15)

Routine

Exercise*	Sets	Repetitions
Superset: Incline dumbbell chest press followed by incline dumbbell fly	2 supersets with 30–45 seconds of rest between (increase poundages on 2nd superset)	12–15 each exercise
Superset: Side lateral raise followed by rear lateral raise	2 supersets with 30–45 seconds of rest between (increase poundages on 2nd superset)	12–15 each exercise
Superset: Dumbbell rowing followed by high-pulley rowing	2 supersets with 30–45 seconds of rest between (increase poundages on 2nd superset)	12–15 each exercise
Superset: Cable curl followed by inner-biceps curl	2 supersets with 30–45 seconds of rest between (increase poundages on 2nd superset)	12–15 each exercise
Superset: Bench dip followed by overhead triceps extension	2 supersets with 30–45 seconds of rest between (increase poundages on 2nd superset)	12–15 each exercise

Aerobics

Follow the above routine with 20–30 minutes of aerobics, such as rowing, stair climbing, stationary cycling, cross-country ski machine, or weighted walking.

TUESDAY/FRIDAY

Emphasis:	Lower-body development, including abdominal work
Warmup:	10 minutes of relaxed walking
Exercise style:	Moderate to heavy weights and low repetitions (6–10)

Routine

Exercise*	Sets	Repetitions
Close-stance half squat	Warmup set (light poundage)	10–12
	2–3 (increase poundage each set)	6–10
Close-stance leg press	Warmup set (light poundage)	10–12
	2–3 (increase poundage each set)	6–10
Leg curl	Warmup set (light poundage)	10–12
	2–3 (increase poundage each set)	6–10
Standing calf raise	1 (light weight)	Work up to 25 or more
Floor crunch	1	Work up to 25 or more
Seated reverse crunch	1	15–20

Aerobics

Follow the above routine with 20–30 minutes of leg-building aerobics, such as Crossrobics or stair climbing.

SATURDAY

Emphasis:	Fat burning

Aerobics

For variety, follow a cross-training aerobics program for 45–60 minutes. Perform 15–20 minutes of 3–4 different types of aerobic exercise. Examples include walking, treadmill walking, stair climbing, Crossrobics, stationary cycling, or rowing. Be sure to cool down with some relaxed walking.

WEDNESDAY/SUNDAY

Rest

---

*If your gym or workout facility does not have certain types of machines or equipment, refer to Appendix C for exercise substitutions.

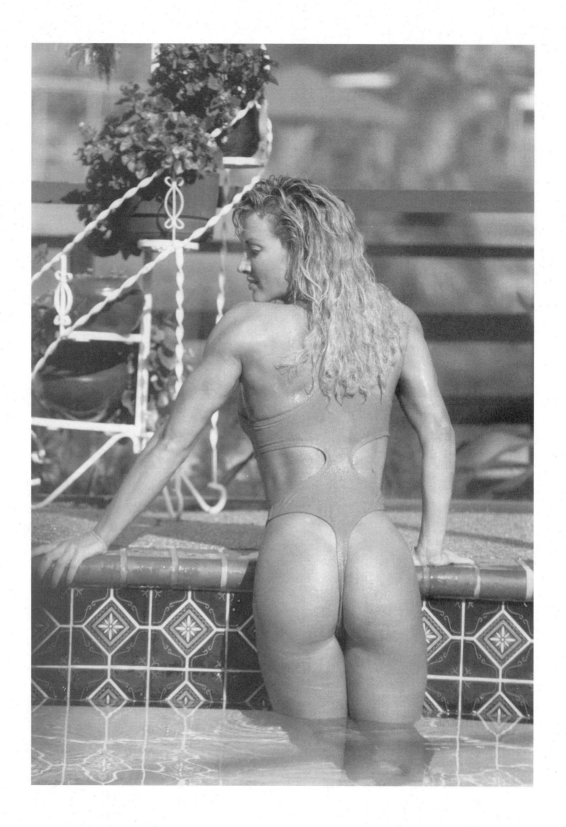

11

The X-Frame: Nearly Perfect, but Always Room for Improvement

Lucky you! Your figure approaches the classic hourglass shape, with your upper body and lower body in equal proportion, tied together by a small waistline. Other possible attributes of an X-frame include arms with balanced development, a bustline just right for your size, and legs that flow aesthetically from the hips to the knees.

But even X-frames have room for improvement! Although you have classic proportions, you may need to trim down. The right diet and aerobics will take care of that. While fighting the fat, you'll use your shape-training routine to firm up the flabby muscle underneath. You'll get back to your hourglass shape in no time.

Preserving Your Shape Even as You Age

A major issue for X-frames—and all body types, really—is preserving your figure as you get older. Body shape tends to change with age. Let's take a look at what happens as the years go by.

As young as your 20s, you begin to lose body-firming muscle. Of course, the best way to prevent that is with exercise, particularly shape training. Fortunately, any body fat you have is distributed rather evenly. Skin is tight and elastic, although on-and-off dieting can compromise this healthy resiliency.

By the time you reach your 30s and 40s, certain factors have begun

Debbie Kruck is definitely an X-frame.

to take their toll: childbearing, gravity (which makes body parts like breasts and buttocks sag), and hormonal changes. These all result in a shifting shape: Muscles are less toned, and excess body fat tends to settle around the hips and thighs.

These changes continue into your 50s and 60s, with others showing up. Aerobic capacity is on the wane. Your bone structure starts to change, with a narrowing of the shoulders and a widening of the pelvis. Body fat begins drifting to the waistline, and the chest begins to shrink. By age 60, your X-frame could look more like an A-frame. Between ages 30 and 70, the average woman typically gains 15 pounds.

Preserving the shape and firmness of your body over time is directly related to muscular development, achieved mainly through weight-training exercises, like those explained in this book, coupled with a healthy diet. What's more, this type of fitness program helps build bone and maintain its integrity, thus minimizing age-related structural changes. Combine shape training with regular aerobics and you'll start reversing declines in aerobic capacity, too. And it's never too late to start.

Shape-Training Exercises for X-Frames

Your shape-training routine is designed to sculpt the body equally, with the goal of firming up and preserving your X-frame. You'll perform a total body workout just three times a week, on nonconsecutive days. Your repetitions are kept in the moderate to high range for toning and overall development.

If you need to knock off fat pounds, keep your rest periods between sets brief (30 seconds), and add an extra set or two to each exercise. Try to perform aerobic exercise five times a week for 30 to 40 minutes each session. Aerobics before breakfast, as well as after your weight training, will help accelerate the fat-burning process. We suggest fast walking, weight walking, racewalking, jogging or running, aerobic dance, or any of the high-tech aerobic exercise options. Following are the shape-training exercises in your routine.

Medium-Stance Hack Squat
Targets: Upper thighs, buttocks, and calves

Step into the hack squat machine and face forward. Place your feet 10 to 12 inches apart, with your toes pointing forward. Release the safety latches, and slide up and down by bending and straightening your knees. In the bent-knee position, your thighs should be parallel with the platform of the machine.

Changing the position of your feet changes the segment of the muscle worked. If you want to work

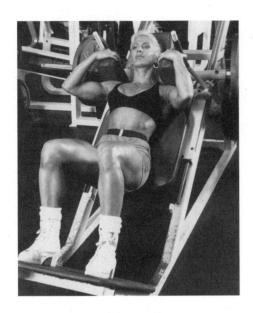

Medium-stance hack squat

your outer thighs, for example, take a wider stance, with your feet placed shoulders' width apart on the platform and your toes angled out. Perform the exercise as instructed.

Dumbbell Side Lunge
Targets: Inner thighs and rear of thighs

Hold a dumbbell in each hand at your sides. Keeping your back as straight as possible, step out to your right side as far as you can until your thigh is just about parallel to the floor. Try to keep your left leg straight. Step back to the starting position. Continue the exercise on your right leg for the suggested number of repetitions. Repeat the exercise with your left leg.

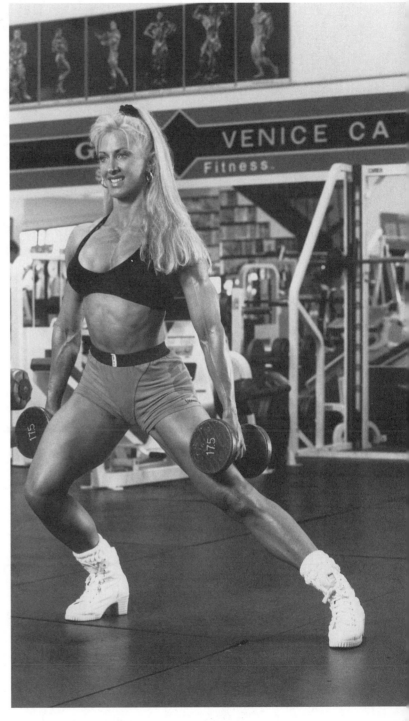

Dumbbell side lunge

is one of the most difficult body spots to develop and tone. This exercise does the trick.

To perform it, you'll need a leg extension machine. Face the seat of the machine, and position yourself between the seat and the padded foot roller. You'll exercise one leg at a time. Place the back lower part of the exercising leg under the foot roller. Grasp the sides of the seat and lean forward slightly. Curl your leg up toward your buttocks. You should feel a deep, muscle-stimulating burn in your buttocks and hamstrings. Lower your leg slowly. Complete your set, then work the other leg.

Machine Bench Press
Targets: Pectoral (chest) muscles

Machine bench presses come in various types of models. In some, you take an upright position and press the bar forward; in others, you lie at an incline or on your back and press the bar upward. Either way, you may have to adjust the seat, the bar, or both to accommodate your height.

Select a weight, and position yourself in the machine. Take hold of the bar and press out, locking your elbows when your arms are fully extended. Slowly return to the starting position. Repeat the exercise for the suggested number of repetitions.

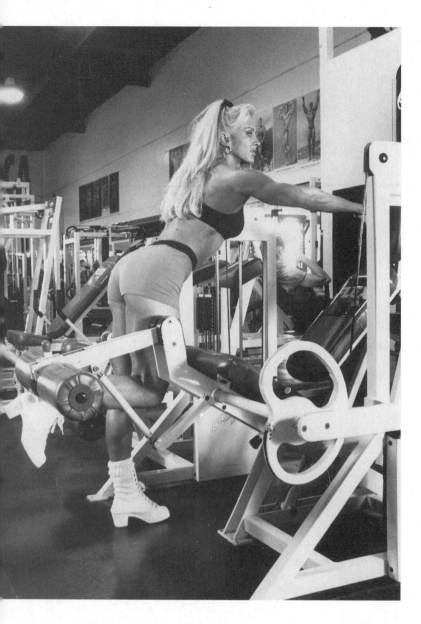

Hip/hamstring curl

Hip/Hamstring Curl
Targets: Hamstrings and buttocks

The point at which the rear of the upper legs meets the lower buttocks

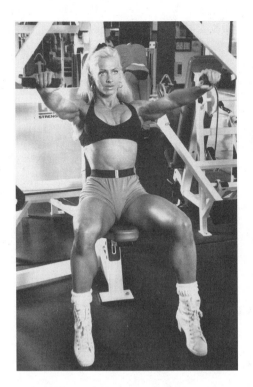

Machine bench press

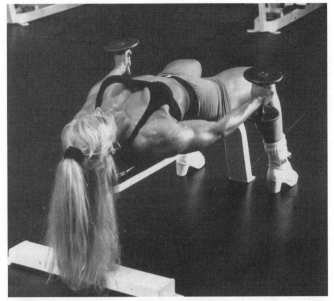

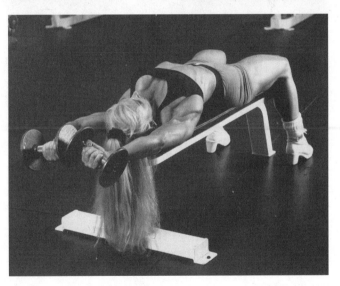

Chest circle

Chest Circle

Targets: Pectoral (chest) muscles

Chest circles are an excellent firming exercise for the chest, especially the outer segments. They also develop flexibility in the upper body.

To begin, take a dumbbell in each hand, and lie back on a flat bench. With the palms of your hands facing inward, hold the dumbbells next to the side of each thigh. The top of each dumbbell should be facing upward. In a circular motion, bring the dumbbells out and around past your midsection and chest until they meet together behind your head. During this movement, turn your hands so that your palms face upward. Return to the starting position, following the same circular path used in the beginning phase of the exercise. Repeat the movement, using the suggested number of repetitions.

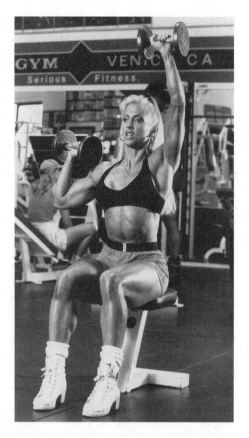

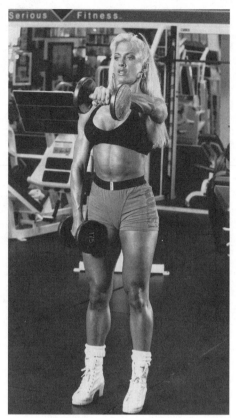

One-Arm-at-a-Time Dumbbell Press
Targets: Front and outer shoulders

Take a dumbbell in one hand, and hold on to a piece of equipment with the other hand for support. Begin with the dumbbell at shoulder level and your palm facing outward. Press the dumbbell up to an overhead position, and lock your elbow at the top. Slowly lower to the starting position. Repeat the exercise for the suggested number of repetitions. Complete your set, then work the other shoulder in the same manner.

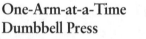

Front lateral raise

Front Lateral Raise
Targets: Front shoulders

To begin, hold a dumbbell in each hand at your sides, palms down, and stand with your feet a comfortable distance apart. Slowly raise the dumbbells straight up in front of your body until they reach eye level. Keep your elbows slightly bent throughout the exercise. Lower slowly. Repeat for the suggested number of repetitions.

Negative Chin-Up
Targets: Upper back

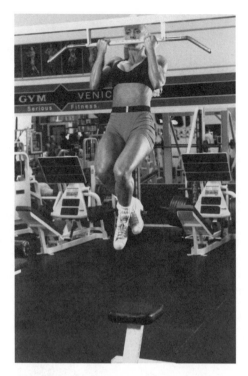

As noted earlier, the conventional chin-up exercise is often too difficult for women to perform because it requires immense upper-body strength. That's too bad, since this exercise is wonderful for keeping the upper back in great shape. Not to worry, though. There's a solution that's equally effective: the negative chin-up. It emphasizes the "negative," or lowering, portion of the chin-up exercise.

Have someone hoist you up to a chinning bar, or use a stool. Some machines, like the Nautilus Omni machine, have steps so you can reach the bar on your own. Either way, take a wide underhand grip on the bar, and position yourself so that your chin is just above the bar. Next, slowly lower your body to a position in which you are hanging at arm's length. Keep your torso steady, without swaying back and forth. After completing this lowering movement, hoist yourself back up to the bar using assistance (a partner, stool, or steps), and repeat the exercise. Do as many repetitions as you can.

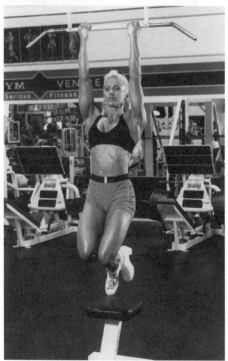

Negative chin-up

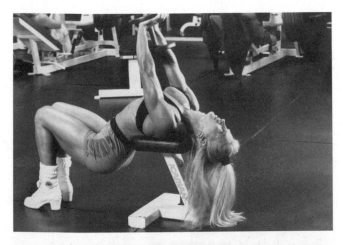

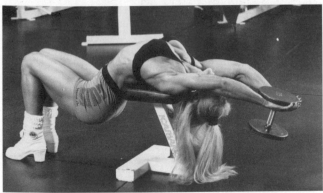

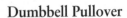

Dumbbell pullover

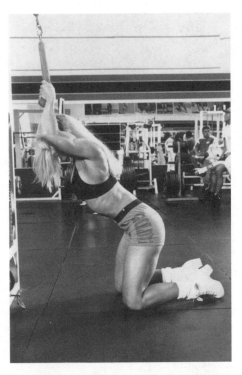

Dumbbell Pullover

Targets: Back, pectoral (chest) muscles, and triceps (back) of upper arm

Grasp a dumbbell at one end with your palms against the inside plate. Position your body crosswise to an exercise bench with your upper back resting on the bench and your knees bent. Bend your elbows slightly, and slowly bring the dumbbell back over your head. Try to get a good stretch in your upper-back muscles. Return

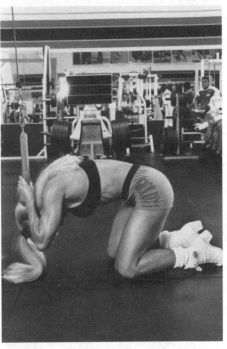

Pulley crunch

the dumbbell to the starting position. Repeat the exercise for the suggested number of repetitions.

Pulley Crunch
Targets: Abdominals

The pulley crunch is a great tightener for the upper and lower abdominals. To begin, select a weight at which you can do up to 25 repetitions. Hold the rope or handle of a high pulley on a cable machine, and kneel facing the machine. Use the strength of your abdominal muscles to curl down to somewhat of a hunched position. Slowly return to the starting position. Repeat the exercise.

Lying Dumbbell Curl
Targets: Biceps of arm

You perform the lying dumbbell curl on a flat exercise bench. Take a dumbbell in each hand, and lie back on the bench. Begin the exercise with your arms extended straight down, with the palms of your hands facing forward. Curl the weights up at your sides in an arc toward your chest. Slowly lower the dumbbells to the starting position. Repeat the exercise for the suggested number of repetitions.

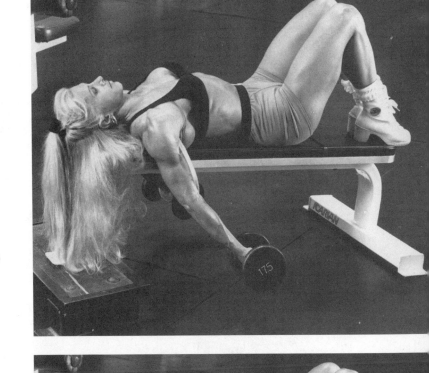

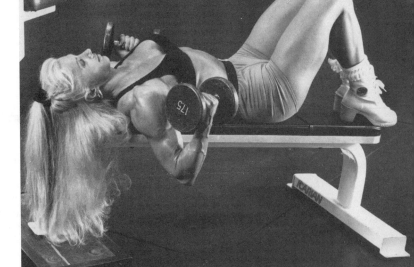

Lying dumbbell curl

THE X-FRAME: NEARLY PERFECT, BUT ALWAYS ROOM FOR IMPROVEMENT   139

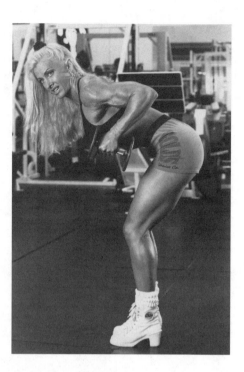
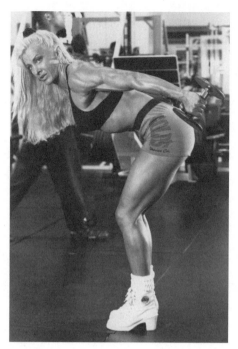

Dumbbell Kickback
Targets: Triceps (back) of upper arm

At the back of your upper arm, the triceps accounts for three-fourths of your muscle, so you want to work your triceps properly. One of the best exercises for keeping this three-part muscle in shape is the dumbbell kickback.

To begin, hold a dumbbell in each hand, and bend forward at the waist until your torso is parallel to the floor. Your legs should be a comfortable distance apart, with knees slightly bent.

Bend your elbows, and press your upper arms to your sides. Press the dumbbells backward in an arc until your arms are fully extended and parallel to the floor. In this position, lock your elbows and squeeze your triceps. Slowly return to the starting position. Repeat the exercise for the suggested number of repetitions.

Calling All Body Types: The X-Frame Routine as Maintenance Shape Training

A goal of all the shape-training routines in this book is to redistribute body weight toward more of an X-frame shape. Once you feel as though you've reached that goal, you can use the X-frame routine to maintain and further hone your new figure.

Shape-Training Routine: X-Frames

MONDAY/WEDNESDAY/FRIDAY

Emphasis:	Maintaining shape or trimming down
Warmup:	5–10 minutes of relaxed walking
Exercise style:	Moderate to heavy poundages and high reps (12–15)

Routine

Exercise*	Sets	Repetitions
Medium-stance hack squat	Warmup set (light weight)	10–12
	2–3 (increase poundage each set)	12–15
Dumbbell side lunge	Warmup set (light weight)	10–12
	2–3 (increase poundage each set)	12–15
Hip/hamstring curl	Warmup set (light weight)	10–12
	2–3 (increase poundage each set)	12–15
Machine bench press	Warmup set (light weight)	10–12
	2–3 (increase poundage each set)	12–15
Chest circle	Warmup set (light weight)	10–12
	2–3 (increase poundage each set)	12–15
One-arm-at-a-time dumbbell press	Warmup set (light weight)	10–12
	2–3 (increase poundage each set)	12–15
Front lateral raise	Warmup set (light weight)	10–12
	2–3 (increase poundage each set)	12–15
Negative chin-up	1 set. Use body weight	As many as possible
Dumbbell pullover	Warmup set (light weight)	10–12
	2–3 (increase poundage each set)	12–15
Pulley crunch	1–2	25–50
Lying dumbbell curl	Warmup set (light weight)	10–12
	2–3 (increase poundage each set)	12–15
Dumbbell kickback	Warmup set (light weight)	10–12
	2–3 (increase poundage each set)	12–15

Aerobics

If you need to burn fat, follow the above exercise routine with 30 to 45 minutes of aerobic exercise. Excellent choices include fast walking, weight walking, racewalking, jogging or running, aerobic dance, or any of the high-tech aerobic exercise options.

TUESDAY/SATURDAY

Emphasis: Fat-burning and cardiovascular fitness

On these non-weight training days, perform 30 to 45 minutes of aerobic exercise. Excellent choices include fast walking, weight walking, racewalking, jogging or running, aerobic dance, or any of the high-tech aerobic exercise options. For fat-burning try to get in five aerobic sessions weekly; for general fitness and cardiovascular health, three aerobic sessions weekly are sufficient.

THURSDAY/SUNDAY

Rest or aerobics

---

*If your gym or workout facility does not have certain types of machines or equipment, refer to Appendix C for exercise substitutions.

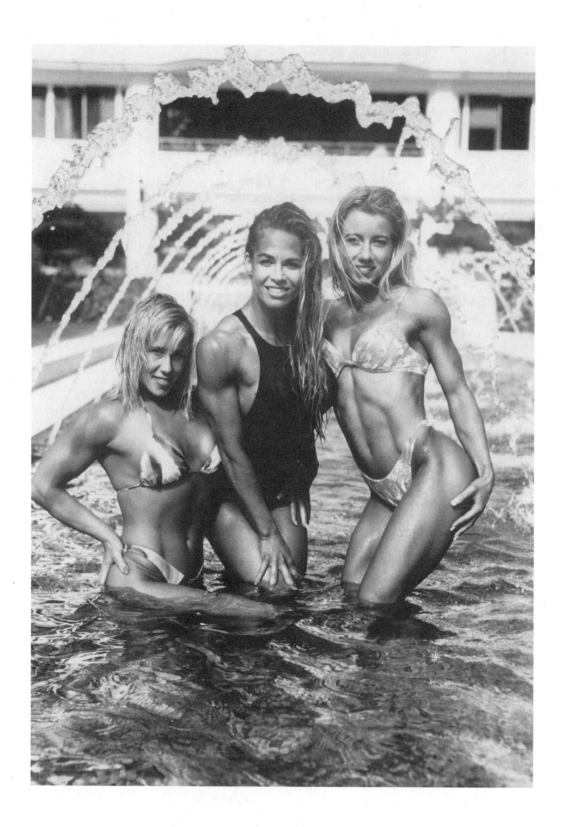

Shape Training at Home

Working out in the comfort of your own home is the best option for millions of people because it has so many advantages. One of the biggest is convenience. You don't have to spend time getting to and from the gym. A home workout better conforms to your schedule.

You can also save money by working out at home. A set of free weights (dumbbells and barbells) costs well under $200, whereas a health club membership may cost anywhere from $250 a year on up. Your weight set will last for years, as long as you take care of it; with a gym membership, you have to pay up annually.

Economics aside, the privacy factor appeals to many women. If you don't like the way you look in gym clothes, no one has to see you exercising at home. You can focus on reshaping your body without feeling inhibited.

How Should I Equip My Home Gym?

If working out at home is your cup of tea, there are four types of equipment to consider purchasing: free weights, generic equipment (benches and mats), multistation weight machines, and aerobic equipment. As you shop around, it's important to know what you're buying—and why.

A typical starter set of free weights contains one barbell rod, two dumbbell rods, collars, and plates totaling 110 pounds or more. Be sure to purchase a set with enough combined weight that you can gradually up your poundages. Challenging your muscles to lift more weight produces the body-changing results you want.

Along with free weights, a good addition to your home gym is a sturdy bench with a rack to hold a barbell. A bench/rack configuration

Fitness models Pepper Ferry, Amy Fadhli, and Candice Head

expands your exercise possibilities. Some benches bend and tilt at the middle so you can do incline or decline exercises, which work the muscles from additional angles. Depending on the product, bench prices usually start at around $100.

Beware of flimsy benches. Look for one that will support you and the potential weight you'll be using. A welded frame constructed with thick tubing will be stronger than one assembled with bolts. Adequate padding is important, too. The best way to judge a bench is to "test-drive" it at the store. If if wiggles, forget it.

To do leg extensions and leg curls, you can purchase special attachments that hook onto your bench. Some of these devices, however, are not designed well enough to fit all body types. So before buying any attachment, try it out.

Exercise mats are a must for the home gym. For abdominal exercises and warmup stretches, they cushion you from the hard floor.

The third type of home weight-training equipment is the multistation weight machine, which is similar to those you find in health clubs but scaled down to fit the home. These versatile units are made up of one or more positions from which different muscle groups can be trained.

The drawbacks of multistation machines are that they take up more room and are more expensive than free weights. Plan on spending between $1,500 and $5,000 for a good one. Prices hinge on the number of exercise stations and quality of construction.

If you can afford a multistation machine, which one should you buy? Plenty are out there. Some employ weight stacks for resistance; others, heavy bands. Some are quite elaborate in design, while others are rather simple. A good rule of thumb to follow is to stick with well-known brands. As with any exercise equipment, first test it out for fit and feel.

For aerobic conditioning and fat burning, you'll need some aerobic equipment. There are several choices for home use: stationary bicycles, rowing machines, treadmills, stair climbers, and cross-country ski machines. You can also get a good aerobic workout by following an exercise video. Make sure the video takes you through at least 20 to 30 minutes of heart-pumping action and that the dance moves are easy to follow.

Are There Home Shape-Training Exercises That Don't Require Equipment?

As you'll see later in this chapter, you can do certain exercises using your own body weight or everyday items like towels, broomsticks, and chairs for resistance. This type of training, called *nonapparatus training*, can be quite effective for increasing muscle tone. Exercising with your own body weight requires balance, and you work more muscles in the process. It requires lots of energy, and the result is a high level of fitness.

Where's the Best Place to Set Up My Home Gym?

Set up your home gym in a room with plenty of space, so you can fit in your equipment. A room that's too crowded can be uncomfortable to exercise in, and it may present too many tripping hazards.

Your exercise room should be well ventilated, too. If your air conditioner doesn't move enough air, keep the air circulating with an electric fan. The optimum temperature range for working out is between 60 and 80 degrees Fahrenheit.

If possible, put up some mirrors in the room to help you check your exercise technique. At home, you can work out in your bra and actually see your muscles being worked. This instant feedback is encouraging.

Perhaps most important, your workout area should be a room you like being in. Many people make the mistake of choosing a dark corner of the garage or a dungeonlike basement. If you do, you won't feel like going in there. As a home weight trainer, you need to maximize everything you can for motivation.

How Can I Stick to My Shape-Training Routine at Home?

No doubt about it, the home exerciser has a tougher time being faithful to her routine. Part of the motivation for those who are members of fitness centers is the chance to socialize at the gym. So the woman on her own needs other motivators. Here are a few pointers:

Keep records of your repetitions, sets, and poundages. Measuring and seeing progress will help keep you going.

Find a picture of a person whose body you admire—someone with a bone structure similar to yours—and keep it where you can see it. Then imagine yourself looking like that person.

If you really need an extra nudge, consider hiring a qualified personal trainer—a fitness professional who comes to your home and guides you through your routine. When you have a personal trainer coming over, it's not that easy to miss a workout. To get results, you need the consistency of regular workouts. A trainer can help you stick to it. A downside of a personal trainer is expense. A trainer costs anywhere from $25 to more than

$100 an hour. But remember, you're making an investment in yourself!

Home Shape-Training Exercises

What follows are exercises and a routine designed for home use. You can also use any barbell or dumbbell exercise explained in this book in home shape training. If you own a home multistation gym, you can include other exercises as well. You can also tailor this core shape-training routine to your body type:

- A-frames should do extra sets (a total of 4 to 5 sets) of leg and buttock exercises, plus aerobics for 30 to 45 minutes five times a week.
- H-frames should include extra sets of abdominal exercises, using other abdominal exercises featured in this book.
- I-frames should follow the routine as described, using heavier weights and low repetitions. If you have a barbell set at home, consider using your barbells in place of the leg, shoulder, and chest exercises in this routine.
- O-frames should strive to do additional sets of all exercises, as well as a higher number of repetitions. Do aerobics for 30 to 45 minutes five times a week.
- T-frames should work on building the lower body by using

heavier weights and low repetitions (6 to 10). If you have a barbell set, use barbell exercises in place of the freehand squat.
- X-frames can use the home shape-training routine without substitutions. Just remember to work out as intensely as possible—advice that goes for all body types.

Freehand Squat
Targets: Legs and buttocks

Stand with your legs a comfortable distance apart and your arms crossed over your chest. Keeping your back straight, squat down until your

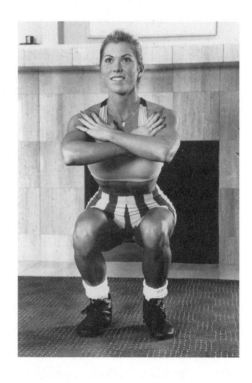

Freehand squat

thighs are just lower than parallel to the floor. Return to the starting position. Repeat the exercise as many times as you can.

Try to keep constant tension on your thighs and buttocks as you perform this exercise.

Dumbbell Squat
Targets: Legs and buttocks

Hold a dumbbell in each hand alongside your body, and stand with your feet a comfortable distance apart. Keeping your back straight, squat down until your thighs are just lower than parallel to the floor. Return to the starting position.

Repeat the exercise as many times as you can.

Try to keep constant tension on your thighs and buttocks as you perform this exercise.

Assisted Leg Curl
Targets: Hamstrings and buttocks

You'll need help from a partner to perform this exercise. Lie facedown on the floor with your legs fully extended. Have your partner place his or her hands on your heels. Curl your legs upward in an arc toward your buttocks while your partner applies resistance as you flex. Next, your partner should try to force your legs back to the starting position as you resist. Repeat both phases of the exercise as many times as you can.

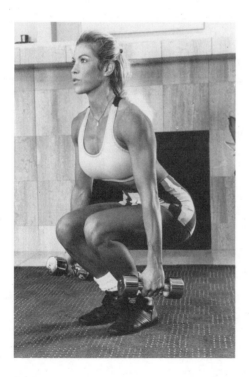

Dumbbell squat

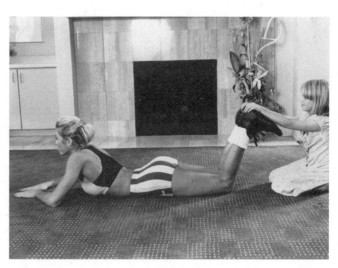

Assisted leg curl

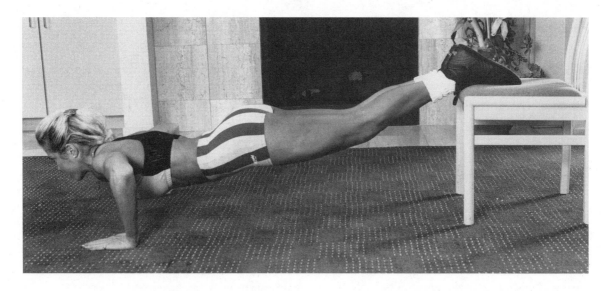

Chair push-up

Chair Push-Up
Targets: Pectoral (chest) muscles

Lie on the floor facedown with your body straight. Elevate your legs by placing the front of your ankles on a chair seat. Position your arms at each side of your chest. Keeping your body straight, press up until your arms are fully extended and your elbows locked. Lower your body slowly to the starting position. Perform as many repetitions as you can.

Concentrate on using the strength of your chest muscles throughout the exercise.

Floor Dumbbell Fly
Targets: Pectoral (chest) muscles

Lie on your back on the floor, and hold a dumbbell in each hand. Begin with your arms stretched out to your sides at shoulder level. Bend your elbows slightly, and bring the dumbbells toward each other in a semicircular movement until they touch over your chest. Slowly return to the starting position. Repeat the exercise as many times as you can.

Lateral Raise
Targets: Shoulders

Use a pair of equally heavy books for the lateral raises. Begin the exercise with the books at your sides, as pictured. Slowly raise them up to a position just above shoulder level. Return slowly to the starting position. Repeat the exercise for as many repetitions as you can.

There's another home version of this exercise that requires a partner. Stand facing your partner with your arms at your sides. Have your partner place his or her hands on your

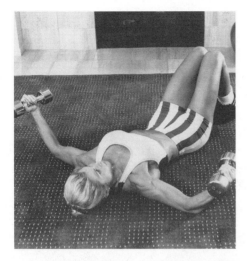 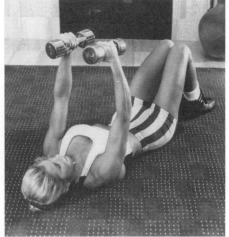

Floor dumbbell fly

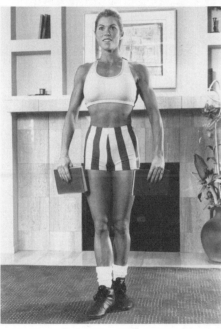 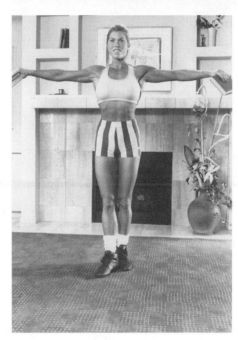

Lateral raise

wrists. Raise your arms upward to a position just above shoulder level while your partner applies resistance. Next, your partner should try to force your arms back to the starting position as you resist. Repeat both phases of the exercise as many times as you can.

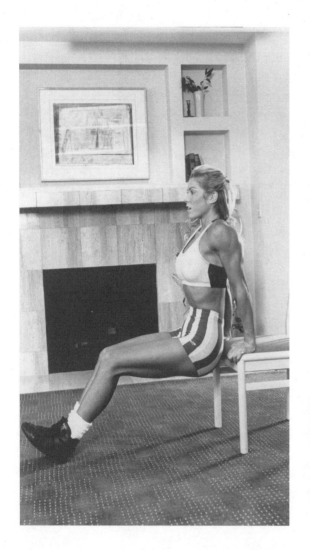
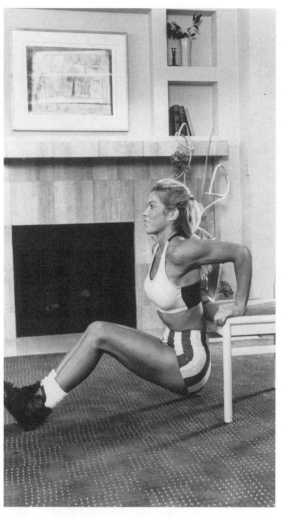

Chair dip

Chair Dip
Targets: Triceps (back) of upper arm

With your back toward a chair, grasp its seat with your hands. Behind your back, your forearms should be facing forward and your fingers pointing toward your feet. Extend your legs and hips forward on the floor so that they form a 45-degree angle with the floor. Slowly bend your elbows, lowering your torso so that your hips are within a few inches of the floor. Once you reach the low position of this movement, press upward again, straightening your arms. Do as many repetitions as you can.

Biceps Curl
Targets: Biceps of arm

Use two heavy books for the biceps curls. To begin, stand with the books at your sides. Flex at the elbow joint, bringing the books upward in an arc toward your shoulders. Slowly return to the starting position. Repeat the exercise for as many repetitions as you can.

Here's another version of this exercise for home use in which you'll need assistance from a partner: Stand facing your partner with your elbows bent, upper arms pressed close to your sides, and palms facing up. Have your partner place his or her hands on the palms of your hands. Curl your lower arms upward in an arc toward your shoulders while your partner applies resistance as you flex. Next, your partner should try to force your arms back to the starting position as you resist. Repeat both phases of the exercise as many times as you can.

Crunch up a Wall
Targets: Abdominal muscles

Lie on your back on the floor, and extend your legs up a wall at a slight angle to the floor. Place your hands behind your head with elbows pointing out. Bend slightly at the waist, using the strength of only your abdominals to bring your upper body toward your legs. Perform as many repetitions as you can.

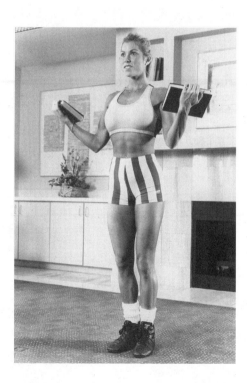

Biceps curl

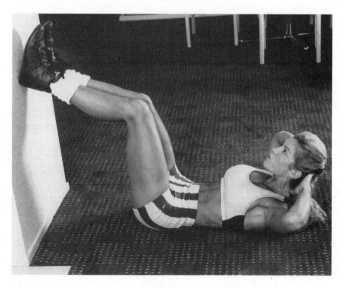

Crunch up a wall

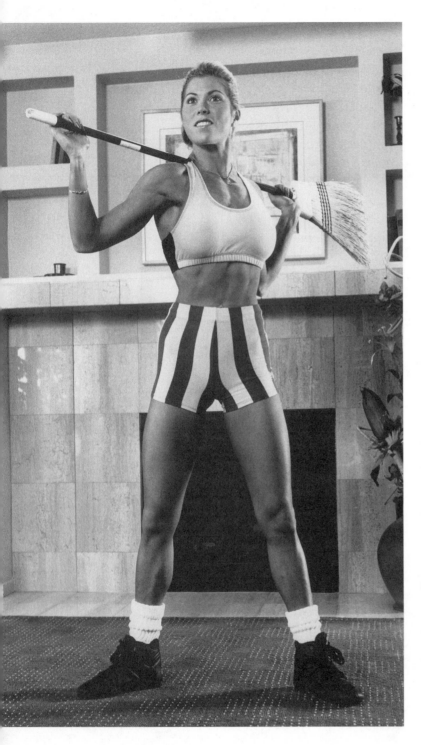

Broomstick Twist
Targets: Abdominal muscles and sides

Place a broomstick or light pole across the rear of your upper back, and hold it there with your hands. Stand with your feet a comfortable distance apart. Twist vigorously from side to side.

Calf Raise on Stairs or Steps
Targets: Calves

Place the balls of your feet on a stair or step so that your heels are just off

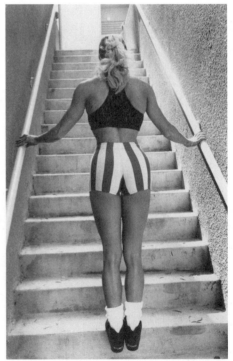

Broomstick twist

Calf raise on stairs

the step. Bend your knees slightly, and hold onto the wall or doorway for support. Raise and lower your heels, getting a good stretch at the bottom of the movement. Do as many repetitions as you can.

The Home Shape-Training Routine

Body Part	Shape-Training Home Exercises	Substitution Exercises for Home Use*
Legs and buttocks	Freehand squat	Barbell squat
	Dumbbell squat	Dumbbell bun burner
Buttocks and hamstrings	Assisted leg curl	Leg curl with bench attachment
		Do-anywhere bun burner
Chest	Chair push-up	Bench press (dumbbell or barbell)
	Floor dumbbell fly	Dumbbell fly on bench
Back		Dumbbell or barbell row
		Pulldown on a home multistation gym
Shoulders	Lateral raise with books or with a partner	Dumbbell lateral raise
		Dumbbell overhead shoulder press
Triceps	Chair dip	Triceps kickback
		Triceps overhead press
Biceps	Biceps curl with books or with a partner	Dumbbell curl
Abdominals	Crunch up a wall	Regular crunch
	Broomstick twist	Dumbbell side bend
Calves	Calf raise on stairs or steps	

*For exercise descriptions, refer to Chapters 6–11.

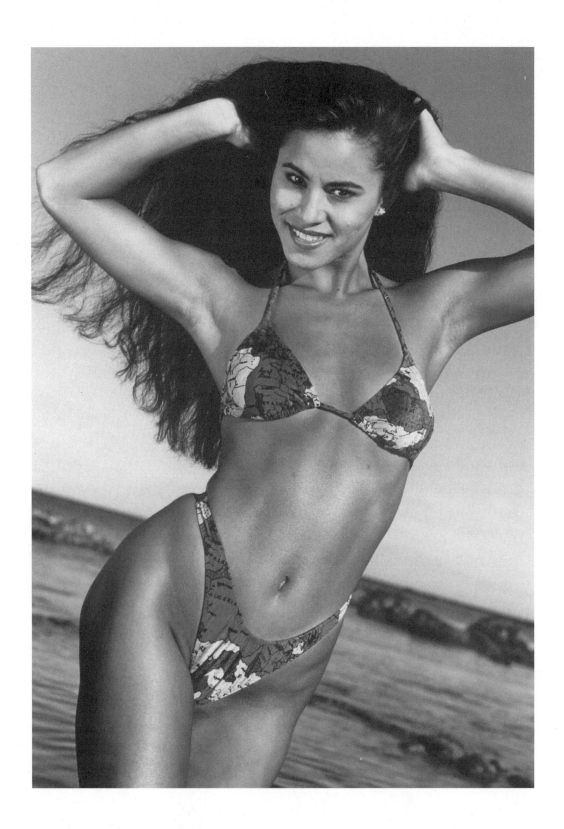

Shape-Training Nutrition

Exercise is one surefire way to take pounds off, as long as you're watching your diet, too. Dieting to lose body fat isn't impossible—all you have to do is make a few minor adjustments.

A 10-Point, Easy-to-Follow Strategy

Here's a dietary strategy to help you whittle away fat painlessly, without deprivation or starvation. It's based on 10 points, each of which is a guideline for successful fat loss.

Point 1: Eat More Calories

Surprise! Low-calorie diets (below 1,200 calories a day) do more harm than good. When calories are in short supply, your body thinks it's starving, and your metabolism slows down. Then your body needs even fewer calories to function. This makes it tougher to continue losing fat and much easier to regain it. Restricting how much you eat simply doesn't work in the long run, since it decreases your ability to burn fat.

Furthermore, in response to low-calorie dieting, a fat-storing enzyme found on the surface of fat tissue goes to work, hoarding fat to protect the body against the effects of starvation. Low-calorie dieting also forces the body to start burning muscle (including heart muscle) for energy, and this lowers your metabolism even more.

The trick is to consume enough calories to keep your metabolism high, but get enough of a caloric deficit to burn fat. Considering that there are 3,500 calories in a pound of fat, how many calories do you need daily to lose fat healthfully?

First, you need to determine your total calorie needs, based on

Proper nutrition is a key component in staying fit. (Model: Angel Teeves)

how active you are. Exercising in the shape-training program puts you in the "active" category. To fuel their energy needs and maintain their weight, active people need about 16 calories per pound of body weight.

Let's say you currently weigh 140 pounds. The math is simple: 140 pounds × 16 calories = 2,240 calories—your intake to stay at your present weight of 140 pounds.

Suppose you want to lose 20 pounds. Cut your calories by 500 a day to about 1,700, and you'd lose a pound a week (500 × 7 = 3,500)—

a slow, safe rate of loss. The slower you lose fat, the better you keep it off.

Exercise is another way to create a caloric deficit. If you wanted to speed up your fat loss, you could do more exercise each week. On average, an hour of exercise burns 300 to 500 calories.

Most active women can lose fat safely and successfully on a caloric intake of 1,500 to 1,800 calories a day. This provides enough calories to fuel your energy needs and meet your nutritional requirements. The

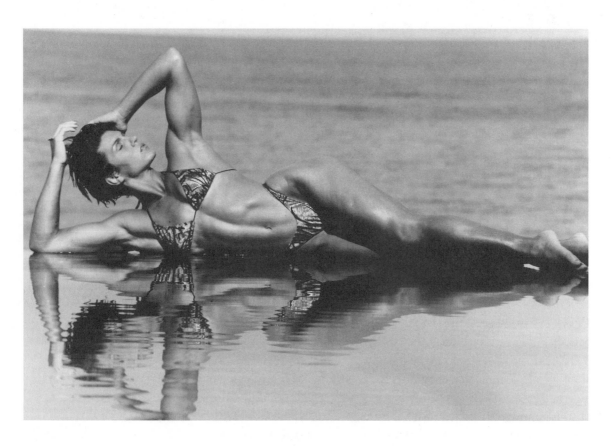

A low-fat diet keeps you in swimsuit shape. (Model: Marjo Selin)

156   SHAPE TRAINING

14-Day Shape-Training Diet described later in this chapter is based on a 1,500-calorie diet.

Point 2: Slash Fat Calories

Fatty foods can fast derail your attempts to shape up. The main reason: Calories from fat (butter, fried foods, cheeses, candy, and so forth) are readily stored as body fat, whereas calories from other foods have to be converted to fat—a process that burns calories.

An easy way to up your fat-burning potential is to cut the fat in your diet. Sometimes that's all you need to do to reduce calories. In one study, a group of women ate as much as they wanted but stuck to low-fat versions of their favorite foods. This low-fat fare automatically cut 220 calories a day from their diets, and the women lost an average of half a pound a week.

Reduce your intake of high-fat foods by sticking to low-fat and nonfat choices: lean proteins like white-meat poultry, fish, and egg whites; low-fat or nonfat dairy products; low-fat salad dressings; and other reduced-fat foods. Learn how to cut the fat from your diet by making healthful substitutions—for example, a baked potato for french fries; skim milk for whole milk; plain yogurt for sour cream or mayonnaise; ice milk or frozen yogurt for ice cream; a grilled chicken sandwich for a cheeseburger; and fat-free pretzels for potato chips. Also, broil,

bake, or microwave foods, rather than frying them.

Watch out for "hidden" fat in certain foods, too. Fat is added to crackers, cookies, breads, and rolls. You may not see it, but it's there.

This all brings up a key point: You need some dietary fat for good health, but how much?

There's some disparity in the scientific community as to how much total fat you should eat daily. Many dietitians and health associations recommend that total fat calories should represent less than 30 percent of your total calories. For losing body fat, other experts suggest going even lower—to 10 or 20 percent of total calories.

Our position is that every person is different, especially since no two metabolisms are exactly alike. Twenty percent of total calories from fat may work perfectly for one person, but not another. You really must find out for yourself. Remember, though, you do need some dietary fat for energy, especially since your body uses fat stores during aerobic activity. Also, fat keeps your joints, skin, and internal organs in good working order.

Point 3: Concentrate on Natural Foods

Natural, unprocessed foods are used more efficiently by the body and are less likely to be stored as body fat. Choose fresh fruits, vegetables, whole grains, and other complex,

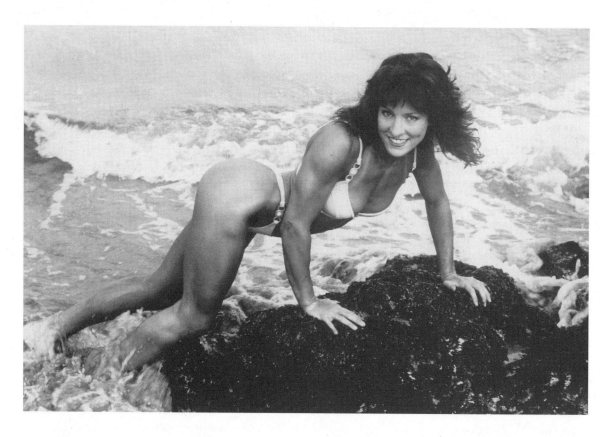

Eating natural foods leads to natural beauty. (Model: Kim Peterson)

natural carbohydrates as the mainstays of your diet.

Natural, complex carbohydrates are required to make and replenish muscle glycogen, the carbohydrate stored in the muscles and liver and used to supply energy for exercise and activity. In fact, research has shown that complex carbohydrates do a better job of this than refined or simple carbohydrates.

Natural foods are also rich in fiber. They contain two types of fiber: soluble and insoluble. Soluble fiber, found in oats, rice bran, dried peas and beans, and prunes, helps lower cholesterol. Good sources of insoluble fiber, which keeps your digestive tract healthy and free from cancer-causing substances, include whole grains, fruits, and vegetables.

Foods like refined pasta and bread products are less effective in a fat-loss program. These foods have undergone too much processing, so your body does not use them as well; they tend to be converted into body fat. If you limit processed foods to no more than a few times a week, you'll notice a huge difference in your body definition and shape.

Point 4: For Faster Fat Loss, Moderate Your Intake of Carbohydrates

As energy foods, carbohydrates are absolutely essential for exercisers and must be included in your diet. But if you want to speed up your fat loss, curtail your carb intake slightly. When you reduce carbohydrates, your body has less glycogen to run on, so it starts burning more fat instead.

There's a drawback, though: A diet low in carbohydrates results in low energy and a cranky mood (because less glucose gets to the brain, and glucose is brain fuel). So what's a body to do?

Here's the solution: Include a complex carb at every meal except dinner. That way, you'll still have enough carbohydrates earlier in the day when you need them the most for exercise and other activities. If your body and mind can stand it, eliminate carbohydrates altogether after midafternoon. Cutting out carbohydrates in the evening reduces the number of calories at dinner. That's good, since a light evening meal is better for fat loss. Save your bigger meals for breakfast and lunch.

Generally speaking, your daily carb intake for fat loss should be 55 to 60 percent of your total caloric intake. Here's how to figure your carb needs on a 1,500-calorie diet:

1. Multiply calorie needs by 60 percent: $1,500 \times .60 = 900$ calories from carbohydrates.
2. Divide 900 by 4, since there are 4 calories in a gram of carbohydrate: $900/4 = 225$ grams of carbohydrate a day.
3. Divide 225 grams by 4 for breakfast, midmorning snack, lunch, and midafternoon snack: $225/4 = 56$ grams of carbohydrate per meal or snack. For the nutrient content of various foods, it's a good idea to have a calorie and gram counter guide on hand.

Once again: Every body is different! You may need even fewer carbs (or more) than the formula states. Let your body and your energy levels be your guide.

Point 5: Limit Sugar Consumption

Sugars—honey, syrup, table sugar, brown sugar—are quickly digested into glucose, a sugar in the blood that is converted into glycogen for the muscles and liver or carried in the blood to fuel the brain and muscles. If you eat too much sugar at once, the excess can be turned into body fat. This happens because excessive sugar triggers a surge of the hormone insulin. Insulin activates certain enzymes that promote fat storage. Natural, complex carbohydrates don't cause this reaction, which is why they're less likely to be stored as fat. So avoid excess sugar if you're fighting fat.

Point 6: Eat Enough Protein

The exercising body requires ample protein to develop and maintain body-firming muscle. In digestion, protein is broken down into subunits called amino acids, which are reshuffled back into protein to make and repair body tissues. Certain amino acids used in building muscle proteins can be burned by the body during exercise, especially intense aerobic workouts. This is one of the main reasons exercisers need a little more protein in their diets than sedentary people. If you don't get enough, your body can start breaking down muscle tissue to get amino acids for energy. Consequently, you'll lose metabolically active muscle and sabotage your fat-loss efforts.

A lot of controversy surrounds exactly how much protein active people should eat, with recommendations ranging from 15 to 25 percent of total calories. Where fat loss is concerned, some of the current thinking indicates that the body needs a daily intake of between 20 and 25 percent of daily calories to maintain muscle while losing fat. We agree with that recommendation, since better muscle definition and shape can be achieved with a moderately high amount of protein in the diet.

As previously illustrated with carbohydrates, here's how to figure your protein needs for a 1,500-calorie diet:

1. Multiply protein needs by 20 percent: $1,500 \times .20 = 300$ calories from protein.
2. Divide 300 by 4, since there are 4 calories in a gram of protein: $300/4 = 75$ grams of protein a day.
3. Divide 75 grams by 3 for at least three meals that include protein (breakfast, lunch, and dinner, although you could have protein with snacks for a total of 5 times a day): $75/3 = 25$ grams of protein per meal.

There are about 25 grams of protein in three ounces of white-meat poultry, fish, and lean meat; 8 grams in a cup of skim milk or nonfat yogurt; 18 grams in a four-ounce serving of tofu; and about 8 grams in a half cup of cooked beans or legumes. If you don't like to fuss with gram counting, just be sure to have a few ounces of protein with each meal and you'll easily satisfy your protein requirement.

Point 7: Vary Your Diet

The time-worn but sage advice to eat a varied diet has taken a modern twist with the discovery of *phytochemicals* in food. Phytochemicals are naturally occurring substances in fruits and vegetables that have a protective effect against cancer, heart disease, and other life-shortening illnesses. They have funny, hard-to-pronounce names like allylic sulfides, genistein, and isothiocyanates. But there are hundreds, maybe thousands, of them in our foods. The greater the variety of foods you eat, the more phytochemicals you get in your diet.

A vegetarian food loaded with phytochemicals is tofu, also one of your best low-fat, nutrient-rich friends when you're trying to lose body fat. The phytochemicals in tofu and other soy products help keep hormones in healthy balance in women. In menopausal women (who have low levels of the hor-

mone estrogen), the phytochemicals can raise estrogen. They also lower estrogen in women who have too much. This normalizing effect helps control uncomfortable menopausal symptoms, and it may reduce the risk of cancers associated with elevated estrogen. Soy-based foods are so important to women's health that we've included tofu and soy milk recipes in our 14-Day Shape-Training Diet.

There's another big advantage to a varied diet: Too many weight-loss diets restrict calories, and thus nutrients, leading to dangerous deficiencies in vitamins and minerals. In chronic dieters, such nutritional bankruptcy causes anemia (iron

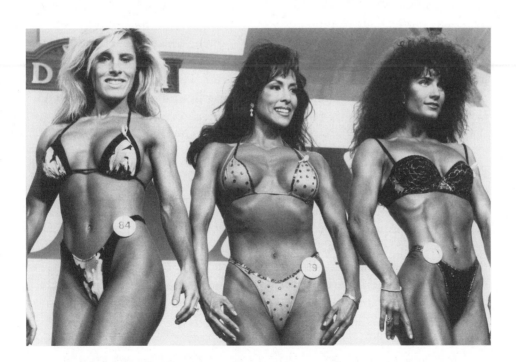

Beautiful bodies are the result of a healthy lifestyle.

deficiency), irregular heartbeat, weakened immune system, fatigue, and headaches, to name just a few problems. By eating lots of nutrient-rich foods, you can head off these problems at the pass.

Which all brings up the question of supplements. Supplements are nothing more than that—supplements. They provide nutrients, vitamins, minerals, and so forth that are already found in food, but usually not in such high concentrations. Some companies make outlandish claims about their products like "burns fat fast" or "builds muscle." The fact is, supplement technology has not come that far—yet.

However, one supplement that makes good nutritional sense is a one-a-day antioxidant vitamin and mineral supplement. The rest of your dollars should be spent on high-quality foods. Food is and always will be the prime building factor in the development of a shapely, toned physique.

Point 8: Eat Five Meals a Day

Gone are the days of three squares only! The new advice is to eat *five* meals. This is probably good news, since most people like to nibble throughout the day anyway. Eating frequently throughout the day has several fat-burning and nutritional advantages:

- *Higher calorie-burn rate*—Every time you eat a meal, your meta-bolic rate goes up as heat is given off to digest and absorb food. By eating five meals a day, you give your metabolism extra opportunities to stay cranked up, and that means more fat-burning power.

- *More energy*—With frequent meals, your body has a constant stream of energy-giving nutrients. When it's time to exercise, you'll be full of pep and ready to go.

- *Better absorption of nutrients*—Eating smaller, more frequent meals helps your body better use vitamins and minerals. Research has shown that a higher percentage of nutrients are absorbed with a series of small meals, compared to two or three large ones.

- *Less temptation*—Eating more often reduces the temptation to stray from your fat-losing nutritional program. When you're eating five times a day, every two to three hours, you're less likely to binge on foods you shouldn't have. Nor do you get hungry or prone to cravings. In short, frequent meals shore up your willpower.

Point 9: Serve Up the Right Portions

A nutritious diet includes the right servings and portions of the following foods every day:

- *Four to five servings of fresh fruits and vegetables*—Examples of a serving are one medium piece of fruit, one cup of raw vegetables, or half a cup of cooked vegetables.

- *Four to six servings of natural, complex carbohydrates*—A serving is half a cup of cooked whole-grain cereal or rice, two rice cakes, two tortillas, or one medium baked potato or sweet potato.
- *At least two servings of low-fat dairy products*—A serving is one cup of skim milk, yogurt, or non-fat cottage cheese, or two ounces of fat-free cheese.
- *Two to three servings of protein-rich foods*—Examples of a serving are two to three ounces of white-meat chicken, fish, or lean red meat; a half cup of cooked beans or legumes; or two egg whites.
- *Fats and oils*—Use these sparingly.

Point 10: Moderate Your Alcohol Usage

Alcoholic beverages are loaded with sugary calories (easily converted into body fat) and low in nutritional value. Plus, when there's alcohol in your system, the liver works overtime to process it and doesn't have adequate time to burn fat. In short, drinking alcohol subtracts from your body's fat-burning power.

Not only that, excessive alcohol use increases your chances of developing heart disease, high blood pressure, liver disease, certain cancers, and nutritional deficiencies, among other health-threatening conditions. If you do drink, limit your intake to no more than a few drinks a week. If you have a lot of body fat to lose, it's best to avoid alcohol altogether until you reach your goal.

The 14-Day Shape-Training Diet

With these principles in mind, we present the 14-Day Shape-Training Diet, which consists of five meals a day: breakfast, lunch, dinner, and snacks at midmorning and midafternoon. The diet is based on 1,500 calories a day to ensure a safe, gradual fat loss. If your loss is slower or faster than one or two pounds a week, you should adjust your caloric level up or down. To add calories, simply increase your portions of complex carbohydrates. Counts for carbohydrates, protein, and fat vary; however, this diet is generally low in fat, high in carbohydrates, and moderately high in protein. Recipes featured in the diet appear in Appendix B.

Be sure to drink eight to ten tall glasses of water daily, too. Drinking water can quash cravings for foods you shouldn't eat. It also keeps you well hydrated for exercise.

At first, you'll drop a lot of weight, which is mostly water, glycogen from the muscles, and some fat. After about two weeks, you'll lose less water and glycogen and more fat. A month or more into your fat-loss program, you may even gain weight. If you've been true to your shape-training program and diet, this gain should be muscle. Muscle weighs more than fat and will show up as a gain on the scales. That's why you should stop relying solely on the scale to check your progress. Instead, keep track of your body fat percentage, look at your physique in the mirror (unclothed), and check the fit of your clothes. If your clothes fit less snugly and you look more defined,

you've lost body fat. Taking your body fat percentage will confirm the loss of body fat.

On the 14-Day Shape-Training Diet, daily menus are designed for variety, so that you get a hefty amount of vitamins, minerals, and phytochemicals for good health. If your schedule is hectic, chances are you dine out frequently. The "Dining Out" table provides at-a-glance guidelines on how to make healthy choices at restaurants. These days, most restaurants cater to health-conscious diners, so it's not that difficult to find low-fat cuisine while dining out.

Dining Out

Restaurant Type	Food Selection
Fast food	• Grilled chicken sandwich, no sauce or mayonnaise; top with lettuce, tomato, or onion • Grilled chicken salad with nonfat salad dressing • Smallest hamburger • Baked potato, plain
Fast food—Mexican	• Light tacos, no sour cream
Fast food—beef	• Sliced roast beef sandwich, no sauce
Fast food—fried chicken	• Barbecue chicken sandwich • Herb-broiled white-meat chicken (remove skin) with green beans and small coleslaw (skip the biscuit)
Steak restaurant	• Grilled chicken, fish, or lean red meat with baked potato (plain) or rice; salad with low-fat dressing
Mexican restaurant	• Light tacos, no sour cream • Taco salad, no sour cream • Chicken fajitas, cooked without oil • Grilled chicken or steak with Mexican rice; salad with low-fat dressing
Asian restaurant	• Moo goo gai pan prepared without sauce, served with steamed rice • Any chicken or shrimp entree with vegetables, prepared without sauce, served with steamed rice
Italian restaurant	• Grilled chicken or baked fish entree, served with a vegetable side dish instead of pasta, and a salad with dressing on the side

Day 1

Breakfast:	½ grapefruit 1 cup Low-Fat, Low-Sugar Granola* 1 cup skim milk 2 egg whites, scrambled
Midmorning Snack:	Fruit Frostie*
Lunch:	3 ounces Italian Grilled Chicken* 1 cup brown rice 1 cup coleslaw tossed with nonfat slaw dressing
Midafternoon Snack:	1 large baked potato with nonfat sour cream
Dinner:	Oven "Fried" Fish* 1 cup salad vegetables with 2 tablespoons salad dressing 1 medium apple

Nutrient Count: 1,521 calories; 208 grams carbohydrate; 73 grams protein; 24 grams fat

Day 2

Breakfast:	½ cantaloupe ½ cup hot oatmeal 1 cup skim milk 2 egg whites, scrambled
Midmorning Snack:	1 cup freshly processed carrot juice (or vegetable juice) 2 rice cakes
Lunch:	1 serving Curried Chicken Salad* 1 medium baked sweet potato 1 medium apple
Midafternoon Snack:	1 cup nonfat, sugar-free lemon yogurt
Dinner:	4 ounces broiled fish fillet with 3 tablespoons cocktail sauce 1 cup green beans 1 cup salad vegetables with 2 tablespoons salad dressing

Nutrient Count: 1,578 calories; 212 grams carbohydrate; 80 grams protein; 26 grams fat

---

*See Appendix B for recipes.

Day 3

Breakfast:	1 cup strawberries
	1 cup hot oatmeal
	2 egg whites, scrambled
Midmorning Snack:	Banana Milkshake*
Lunch:	1 serving Tuna Salad Niçoise*
Midafternoon Snack:	Fruit Frostie*
Dinner:	3 ounces baked turkey
	1 cup broccoli
	1 cup corn

Nutrient Count: 1,329 calories; 165 grams carbohydrate; 85 grams protein; 24 grams fat

Day 4

Breakfast:	½ grapefruit
	1 Lean Breakfast Muffin*
	1 cup skim milk
Midmorning Snack:	Banana Milkshake*
Lunch:	1 serving Mediterranean Salad*
Midafternoon Snack:	1 cup vegetable juice
	2 rice cakes
Dinner:	4 ounces round steak
	1 cup brussels sprouts
	½ cup corn

Nutrient Count: 1,485 calories; 160 grams carbohydrate; 80 grams protein; 42 grams fat

Day 5

Breakfast:	1 medium peach
	1 cup Low-Fat, Low-Sugar Granola*
	1 cup skim milk
	2 egg whites, scrambled
Midmorning Snack:	1 cup freshly processed carrot juice or vegetable juice
	2 rice cakes

---

*See Appendix B for recipes.

Lunch:	Two-Minute Tacos*
	1 cup corn
	1 medium apple
Midafternoon Snack:	1 cup skim milk
	2 Natural Muffins*
Dinner:	Grilled chicken salad from a fast-food restaurant, with fat-free salad dressing

Nutrient Count: 1,616 calories; 230 grams carbohydrate; 76 grams protein; 22 grams fat

Day 6

Breakfast:	1 cup blackberries
	1 slice Fat-Free, High-Fiber Apricot Bread*
	1 cup skim milk
	2 egg whites, scrambled
Midmorning Snack:	1 Banana Milkshake*
Lunch:	3 ounces tuna fish
	2 rice cakes
	1 cup vegetable medley (corn, carrots, and peas)
	1 medium orange
Midafternoon Snack:	1 large baked potato with nonfat sour cream
Dinner:	5 ounces steamed shrimp with 3 tablespoons cocktail sauce
	1 cup salad vegetables with salad dressing

Nutrient Count: 1,439 calories; 176 grams carbohydrate; 82 grams protein; 23 grams fat

Day 7

Breakfast:	1 medium apple
	2 Natural Muffins*
	2 egg whites, scrambled
Midmorning Snack:	Fruit Frostie*
Lunch:	3 ounces baked turkey
	1 cup vegetable medley (corn, carrots, and peas)
	1 medium orange

*See Appendix B for recipes.

Midafternoon Snack:	1 cup nonfat, sugar-free vanilla yogurt
	2 rice cakes
Dinner:	Chicken Parmesan*
	1 cup cauliflower
	1 cup coleslaw with nonfat slaw dressing
	1 large baked potato

Nutrient Count: 1,421 calories; 222 grams carbohydrate; 89 grams protein; 16 grams fat

Day 8

Breakfast:	½ grapefruit
	1 cup hot oatmeal
	1 cup skim milk
	2 egg whites, scrambled
Midmorning Snack:	2 rice cakes
	2 slices turkey ham with hot mustard
Lunch:	4 ounces Italian Grilled Chicken*
	1 cup salad vegetables with nonfat salad dressing
	½ cup whole-wheat pasta
	1 medium peach
Midafternoon Snack:	1 slice Fat-Free, High-Fiber Apricot Bread*
	1 cup nonfat, sugar-free vanilla yogurt
Dinner:	Dinner at a Mexican restaurant:
	4 ounces grilled steak
	1 cup Mexican rice
	1 cup salad vegetables with nonfat ranch dressing

Nutrient Count: 1,603 calories; 175 grams carbohydrate; 89 grams protein; 35 grams fat

---

*See Appendix B for recipes.

Day 9

Breakfast:	1 cup strawberries
	1 cup hot oatmeal
	2 egg whites, scrambled
Midmorning Snack:	Banana Milkshake*
Lunch:	3 ounces tuna fish
	2 rice cakes
	1 cup salad vegetables with low-fat salad dressing
	1 medium peach
Midafternoon Snack:	1 cup nonfat, sugar-free lemon yogurt
	2 Natural Muffins*
Dinner:	Oven "Fried" Fish*
	1 cup broccoli
	1 medium baked sweet potato

Nutrient Count: 1,504 calories; 222 grams carbohydrate; 81 grams protein; 16 grams fat

Day 10

Breakfast:	½ cup blueberries cooked with
	1 cup hot oatmeal
	1 cup skim milk
	2 egg whites, scrambled
Midmorning Snack:	Shape-Training Nutrition Bar*
Lunch:	1 serving Curried Chicken Salad*
	1 medium baked sweet potato
	1 medium apple
Midafternoon Snack:	1 cup nonfat, sugar-free vanilla yogurt
	1 medium orange
Dinner:	Tofu Roll-Ups*
	1 cup salad vegetables with salad dressing

Nutrient Count: 1,655 calories; 225 grams carbohydrate; 95 grams protein; 29 grams fat

---

*See Appendix B for recipes.

Day 11

Breakfast:	¹/₂ grapefruit
	1 slice Fat-Free, High-Fiber Apricot Bread*
	1 cup skim milk
	2 egg whites, scrambled
Midmorning Snack:	Fruit Frostie*
Lunch:	Low-Fat Mini Pizzas*
	1 cup salad vegetables with low-fat Italian dressing
Midafternoon Snack:	2 ounces tuna fish
	2 rice cakes
Dinner:	Chicken Broccoli Orientale*
	1 cup brown rice

Nutrient Count: 1,598 calories; 241 grams carbohydrate; 79 grams protein; 15 grams fat

Day 12

Breakfast:	1 cup freshly processed carrot juice or vegetable juice
	1 cup skim milk
	1 cup hot oatmeal
	2 egg whites, scrambled
Midmorning Snack:	Shape-Training Nutrition Bar*
Lunch:	2 ounces baked chicken, cut in strips and served on a large bed of romaine lettuce with 1 onion, chopped, and 2 tablespoons Caesar salad dressing
	¹/₂ cup whole-wheat pasta with 2 tablespoons of non-fat Parmesan cheese
Midafternoon Snack:	1 cup nonfat, sugar-free vanilla yogurt
	¹/₂ cup unsweetened applesauce
Dinner:	4 ounces grilled round steak
	1 cup corn
	1 cup broccoli

Nutrient Count: 1,556 calories; 195 grams carbohydrate; 87 grams protein; 32 grams fat

---

*See Appendix B for recipes.

Day 13

Breakfast:	½ grapefruit 1 cup Low-Fat, Low-Sugar Granola* 1 cup skim milk 2 egg whites, scrambled
Midmorning Snack:	Shape-Training Nutrition Bar*
Lunch:	Two-Minute Tacos* 1 cup corn
Midafternoon Snack:	1 cup nonfat, sugar-free vanilla yogurt 1 medium apple
Dinner:	Dinner at a seafood restaurant: 4 ounces grilled salmon Salad bar with nonfat dressing 1 large baked potato, plain

Nutrient Count: 1,638 calories; 227 grams carbohydrate; 79 grams protein; 25 grams fat

Day 14

Breakfast:	1 cup orange juice 1 serving hot corn grits 1 cup skim milk 2 egg whites, scrambled
Midmorning Snack:	Banana Milkshake*
Lunch:	Grilled chicken salad from a fast-food restaurant, with nonfat salad dressing 1 large baked potato, plain
Midafternoon Snack:	1 slice turkey ham 1 rice cake Hot mustard (optional)
Dinner:	Quick Catfish Creole* 1 cup brown rice 1 cup broccoli

Nutrient Count: 1,366 calories; 192 grams carbohydrate; 76 grams protein; 13 grams fat

---

*See Appendix B for recipes.

Gaining Fat-Free, Quality Weight: Guidelines for I-Frames

The key to gaining shapely weight is to follow the routine outlined for I-frames in Chapter 8—but only as long as you increase your food intake, too. Most nutritionists advise increasing calories by a few hundred a day. It takes roughly 2,500 calories to build a pound of muscle, so conceivably you could gain a pound a week by eating an extra 350 calories a day. Those calories should come from nutrient-rich foods, however, not from sugar and fat-laden junk foods like milkshakes and ice cream. Calories should be increased primarily from natural, complex carbohydrates and secondarily from lean, first-class proteins. Your shape-training routine can then convert those extra calories into added muscle.

Here are some guidelines for gaining fat-free, healthy weight through good nutrition:

Eat five or more meals a day consistently. That way, you'll be constantly supplying your body with the nutrients it needs to develop fat-free muscle.

Eat more complex carbohydrates. Most of your increased portions should come from complex carbohydrates, which supply the energy you need to work out even harder on your shape-training routine. If you've been eating one serving of oatmeal at breakfast, double

up and eat two. The same goes for other meals.

I-frames often have fast-burning metabolisms, which do best on high-carb diets. Consider upping your daily carbohydrates to 70 percent of total daily calories. You can still follow the 14-Day Shape-Training Diet; simply increase your portions.

Consider weight-gain supplements. Protein powders and sports nutrition bars are excellent calorie-dense foods, meaning they're loaded with nutritious, high-grade calories. On average, they provide between 250 and 350 calories per serving—roughly the extra you need each day for muscle building. These supplements are an easy way to provide extra calories, and you can take them with meals or as snacks. If you use these on a regular basis, you're sure to see progress. A word of caution: Don't substitute them for regular foods and meals. They're designed to work hand in hand with a nutrient-rich diet.

In Appendix B, you'll find a delicious recipe for a sports nutrition bar. Commercially, these bars are often expensive, often as much as $2.50 per bar. Ours will cost you practically pennies.

A Final Note

The changes you'll experience from shape training won't happen overnight, but they will happen more rapidly than with other programs you may have tried. But to ensure rapid progress, you must supply the consistency. Stick to your routine without fail, and you'll be rewarded with a body that looks good in whatever you wear and feels good whatever you do.

Appendix A:

Shape Training During Pregnancy

If you're expecting, should you continue your shape-training program? If so, what exercises should you do? Which should you avoid? And how hard should you work out?

Increasingly, medical experts agree that muscle-strengthening exercise and aerobics are safe for mothers-to-be, as long as you know the potential risks and take a common-sense approach when selecting exercises and training intensities. Still, if you're pregnant or planning to be, consult your doctor before starting or continuing any exercise program.

One of the best sources of information on exercise during pregnancy and after the baby is born is the American College of Obstetricians and Gynecologists (ACOG). This organization has established guidelines for exercise during pregnancy and postpartum. These guidelines do not specifically mention weight training, but they address important safety considerations for any exercise program.

Here's some of what you need to know to shape-train safely while baby is on the way:

Joint Laxity
A loosening of the joints occurs during pregnancy. The output of the hormone relaxin increases, allowing the ligaments to soften and stretch in preparation for delivery. Depending on individual responses, your joints may become less stable and therefore more susceptible to soft-tissue injury. As a result, you must choose exercises carefully.

Exercise Selection and Intensity
To prevent injuries to soft tissues, be cautious with compound exercises such as squats or dead lifts—especially after the second trimester, when relaxin production is at its highest. You can still do these

exercises, but definitely lighten your weights. If compound exercises feel uncomfortable, switch to dumbbell or machine exercises that isolate one muscle group at a time.

During pregnancy your goal should be to maintain the levels of fitness you achieved before pregnancy. In other words, don't push it! Your intensity should be moderate—for example, two to three sets of 10 repetitions with weights that are about 60 to 80 percent of the maximum weight you can lift for one repetition. Consider dropping your weights to poundages that will merely preserve your strength and tone. In addition, expectant mothers who have never exercised before should not start during pregnancy.

Exercise Frequency
Work out three times a week or more on a regular schedule, rather than exercising intermittently, to build and/or maintain fitness levels. Irregular patterns of exercise are stressful to the body.

Proper Breathing
Don't hold your breath while exercising. This is always important, but especially so during pregnancy. By holding your breath, you could cut vital oxygen flow to the fetus.

Exercise Position
Exercising while lying on your back is risky, especially after the fourth month of pregnancy. This position can reduce blood supply to the fetus. Many of the shape-training exercises in this book can be performed from a seated or inclined position.

Body Temperature
Exercise increases body temperature—a condition that threatens the health of the fetus. Your temperature should not exceed 100 degrees Fahrenheit (38 degrees Celsius). As a precaution, don't work out in heat or humidity or wear clothing that's too warm.

Aerobic Guidelines
During pregnancy, be especially careful to monitor your heart rate while exercising. According to ACOG, it should not exceed 140 beats a minute, which reflects 60 to 70 percent of maximum aerobic capacity for women of childbearing years. ACOG also suggests that exercising mothers-to-be limit strenuous activity to 15 minutes in duration. Always warm up and cool down before and after exercising.

Choose a safe form of aerobics. Workouts such as aerobic dance, bench step classes, or slide exercising could result in loss of balance, so you should avoid these while pregnant. Swimming and waterwalking are particularly good aerobic choices for expectant mothers who have not exercised much before their pregnancy.

Hydration

To prevent dehydration, drink plenty of water and other fluids before, during, and after exercise. Proper hydration is essential for any active woman, pregnant or not.

Warning Signs

Throughout your pregnancy, listen to your body. If any of the following unusual symptoms appear, stop exercising and call your doctor at once: pain, bleeding, dizziness or faintness, shortness of breath, irregular heartbeat, absence of fetal movement, or other untoward reactions.

For more information on exercising during pregnancy and after your baby is born, contact ACOG at (202) 484-3321.

Appendix B:

Shape-Training Recipes

Cereal, Muffins, Quick Breads

Low-Fat, Low-Sugar Granola

2½ cups apple juice

½ cup reduced-calorie pancake syrup (fructose-sweetened)

2 teaspoons vanilla

14 cups rolled oats

1 6-ounce package dried apricots, chopped

2 tablespoons cinnamon

2 teaspoons nutmeg

Preheat oven to 325°F. In a large saucepan, heat apple juice, syrup, and vanilla to boiling and then remove from heat. Stir in oats and apricots and moisten thoroughly. Mix in cinnamon and nutmeg.

Spray three cookie sheets with nonstick cooking spray. Spread oat mixture onto the sheets and spray the mixture with cooking spray three times to coat it. Bake until dry and crisp—about 50 minutes. Stir the mixture frequently during baking.

Remove from oven. Let cool and pack in airtight containers. The granola does not need refrigeration.

Makes 14 1-cup servings.

Nutrient count per serving: 200 calories; 35 grams carbohydrate; 5 grams protein

Lean Breakfast Muffin

1 English muffin

2 egg whites

1 slice low-fat turkey ham

2 tablespoons fat-free mozzarella cheese

Lightly toast English muffin. Place turkey ham on top of one side; cheese on the other. Broil for about a minute or until cheese has melted.

Scramble egg whites in a pan sprayed with nonstick cooking spray. Place egg whites on turkey ham, and top with remaining English muffin half to form a sandwich.

Makes 1 serving.

Nutrient count per muffin:
222 calories; 27 grams carbohydrate; 23 grams protein; 2 grams fat

Natural Muffins

1 cup oatmeal flour (Blend rolled oats in a blender until fine.)
1 cup cornmeal
1 tablespoon baking powder
$\frac{1}{2}$ teaspoon salt
3 egg whites
2 tablespoons honey
3 tablespoons canola oil
1 cup skim milk

Preheat oven to 400°F. Mix together oatmeal flour, cornmeal, baking powder, and salt. In a separate bowl, blend the remaining ingredients and pour into the dry mixture. Blend thoroughly.

Pour batter into muffin tins that have been sprayed with nonstick cooking spray or into cupcake papers. Bake for 20 to 25 minutes or until a toothpick inserted into a muffin comes out clean.

Makes 1 dozen muffins, which can be served at breakfast, for snacks, or at other meals.

Nutrient count per muffin:
120 calories; 18 grams carbohydrate; 4 grams protein; 4 grams fat

Fat-Free, High-Fiber Apricot Bread

$1\frac{1}{2}$ cups oatmeal flour (Blend rolled oats in a blender until fine.)
1 tablespoon baking powder
1 teaspoon baking soda
$\frac{1}{2}$ teaspoon salt
1 teaspoon cinnamon
$1\frac{1}{2}$ cups wheat bran
1 6-ounce package dried apricots, chopped
$\frac{1}{2}$ cup unsweetened applesauce
1 cup boiling water
2 egg whites
$\frac{1}{2}$ cup reduced-calorie pancake syrup (fructose-sweetened)
1 teaspoon vanilla

Stir together oatmeal flour, baking powder, baking soda, salt, and cinnamon. In a separate bowl, combine bran, apricots, applesauce, and water. Stir well. In another bowl, blend egg whites, syrup, and vanilla. Add bran mixture and egg mixture to the dry ingredients and blend well.

Pour batter into a loaf pan that has been coated with nonstick cooking spray. Bake 1 hour or until a toothpick inserted into the center comes out clean. Remove from oven and let cool. Remove bread from pan and slice.

Makes 12 slices.

Nutrient count per slice:
104 calories; 22 grams carbohydrate; 3 grams protein

Snacks

Fruit Frostie

1 8-ounce container nonfat, sugar-
    free vanilla yogurt
1/3 cup skim milk
1/2 cup frozen berries (blackberries,
    raspberries, or strawberries)

Place all ingredients in a blender,
and puree until smooth. Pour
mixture into a tall glass, and eat
with a spoon.

Makes 1 serving.

Nutrient count per serving:
169 calories; 30 grams
carbohydrate; 12 grams protein

Banana Milkshake

1/2 banana
1 cup carob-flavored soy milk
1 teaspoon instant coffee

Slice banana half, and freeze slices.
Place all ingredients in a blender,
and puree until smooth. Pour
mixture into a tall glass.

Makes 1 serving.

Nutrient count per serving: 214
calories; 40 grams carbohydrate;
6 grams protein; 4 grams fat

Shape-Training Nutrition Bar

3 1/2 cups rolled oats
1 1/2 cups powdered nonfat milk
1 tablespoon cinnamon
1 cup reduced-calorie pancake syrup
    (fructose-sweetened)
2 egg whites
1/4 cup orange juice
1 teaspoon vanilla

Preheat oven to 325°F. Combine
oats, milk powder, and cinnamon in
a bowl, and mix well. In a separate
bowl, beat together syrup, egg
whites, orange juice, and vanilla.
Add to dry mixture, and mix well.

Pour batter into a cookie
sheet that has been sprayed with
nonstick cooking spray. Shape into
a rectangle so that the batter is
approximately 1/4-inch thick. Precut
the batter into 10 rectangular bars.
Bake until brown.

Remove from oven and let cool.
Store in an airtight container.
Nutrition bars need not be
refrigerated.

Makes 10 nutrition bars.

Nutrient count per bar:
130 calories; 20 grams
carbohydrate; 7 grams protein;
0 grams fat (higher in carbohydrates
and protein than commercial
products with a comparable level
of calories)

Vegetarian Entrees

Two-Minute Tacos

1 15-ounce can black beans,
  undrained
1 4-ounce can green chiles,
  undrained
6 taco shells
6 tablespoons salsa

Heat black beans and chiles with their liquid in a saucepan. Remove from heat and drain juices. Spoon bean mixture into taco shells. Top each taco with 1 tablespoon salsa.

Makes 2 servings.

Nutrient count per serving:
370 calories; 55 grams
carbohydrate; 13 grams protein;
10 grams fat

Mediterranean Salad

½ cup canned garbanzo beans,
  drained
2 ounces feta cheese, crumbled
½ medium onion, chopped
½ red bell pepper, chopped
Romaine lettuce
1 tablespoon Italian salad dressing

Arrange beans, cheese, onion, and red pepper on a bed of lettuce. Drizzle with salad dressing.

Makes 1 serving.

Nutrient count per serving:
543 calories; 31 grams
carbohydrate; 16 grams protein;
23 grams fat

Tofu Roll-Ups

10 lasagna noodles
1 pound soft tofu
2 egg whites
¼ cup plus 3 tablespoons nonfat
  Parmesan cheese
1 cup shredded nonfat mozzarella
  cheese
1 tablespoon dried basil
2 teaspoons dried oregano
1 teaspoon garlic salt
¼ teaspoon ground red pepper
¼ teaspoon freshly ground black
  pepper
1 26¾-ounce can light spaghetti
  sauce

Preheat oven to 350°F. Cook lasagna according to package directions.

In a mixing bowl, blend tofu, egg whites, ¼ cup Parmesan cheese, mozzarella cheese, and seasonings until the mixture resembles a paste. Spread out lasagna on aluminum foil. Spread 3 tablespoons tofu mixture on a noodle, up to the edge. Repeat with other noodles. Roll up each noodle, and cut each roll in half.

Fill a 9" × 13" × 2" baking dish with spaghetti sauce. Place lasagna rolls in dish. Sprinkle with 3 tablespoons Parmesan cheese. Cover and bake 45 minutes.

Makes 5 servings.

Nutrient count per serving:
412 calories; 56 grams
carbohydrate; 38 grams protein;
7 grams fat

Meat, Poultry, Fish Entrees

Low-Fat Mini Pizzas

4 English muffins, split into halves
Crushed red pepper
2 slices turkey ham, sliced into small
 pieces
1 cup nonfat spaghetti or pizza
 sauce
1¼ cups shredded nonfat mozzarella cheese

Place muffin halves on a baking
sheet. Sprinkle each half lightly with
crushed red pepper. Top with pieces
of turkey ham. Spread with sauce.
Top with cheese. Broil about 5
minutes or until cheese has melted.

Makes 4 servings.

Nutrient count per serving:
224 calories; 32 grams
carbohydrate; 15 grams protein;
2 grams fat

Curried Chicken Salad

1 package (about 1 pound) skinless
 chicken breasts, baked or boiled
1 6-ounce can unsweetened pineapple juice
4 tablespoons raisins
½ cup boiling water
1 medium onion, finely chopped
1 medium carrot, grated
1 tablespoon curry powder
½ teaspoon salt
¼ teaspoon ginger
5 tablespoons nonfat, sugar-free
 vanilla yogurt
Romaine lettuce

In a microwave-safe dish, pour
pineapple juice over chicken. Cover
and microwave on high for 1
minute. Turn pieces over and rotate
dish. Microwave on high for
another minute. Let chicken stand
5 minutes.

In a small bowl, pour boiling
water over raisins to plump them
up. Set aside.

Remove chicken from dish,
reserving 2 tablespoons juice. Cut
chicken into bite-sized pieces, and
place in a large bowl with onion
and carrot. Drain raisins and add to
bowl. Stir in spices, reserved
pineapple juice, and yogurt. Mix
well.

Chill 2 hours or longer. Serve on
leaves of romaine lettuce.

Makes 4 servings.

Nutrient count per serving:
179 calories; 20 grams
carbohydrate; 21 grams protein;
4 grams fat

Chicken Parmesan

2 cups Corn Chex cereal
¾ cup nonfat Parmesan cheese
3 egg whites
½ cup skim milk
1 package (about 1 pound) skinless
 chicken breasts

Preheat oven to 400°F. Blend cereal
in a blender until fine. Transfer to a
mixing bowl, and stir in Parmesan
cheese. Set aside.

In a small bowl, beat egg whites
and skim milk until well blended.

Dip chicken breasts into egg mixture, then roll in cereal/cheese mixture, coating both sides.

Spray a cookie sheet several times with nonstick cooking spray. Spread chicken breasts on cookie sheet. Lightly coat chicken with spray. Bake 25 minutes.

Makes 4 servings.

Nutrient count per serving: 211 calories; 18 grams carbohydrate; 28 grams protein; 5 grams fat

Italian Grilled Chicken

1 package (about 1 pound) skinless chicken breasts
1 16-ounce bottle fat-free or low-fat Italian salad dressing

Place chicken breasts in a glass dish. Pour salad dressing over chicken. Refrigerate for several hours.

Grill chicken, basting with salad dressing.

Makes 4 servings.

Nutrient count per 4 oz. serving: 100 calories; 20 grams protein; 3 grams fat

Chicken Broccoli Orientale

2 tablespoons cornstarch
1/4 cup plus 2 tablespoons soy sauce
1 package (about 1 pound) skinless chicken breasts, cubed
1/4 cup white wine
4 teaspoons brown sugar
2 teaspoons cider vinegar
2 tablespoons vegetable oil
2 teaspoons crushed red pepper
1 tablespoon chopped garlic
2 medium onions, cut into chunks
1 16-ounce bag frozen broccoli cuts

Blend cornstarch and 1/4 cup soy sauce in a medium bowl. Add chicken and stir to coat. In a small bowl, mix remaining 2 tablespoons soy sauce with wine, brown sugar, and vinegar. Set aside.

Heat oil in a wok at 300°F, and add red pepper and garlic. Cook 1 minute. Add chicken. Stir-fry until chicken is cooked. Add onion and broccoli. Cover wok and cook mixture until broccoli is tender, about 5 minutes, stirring occasionally. Remove cover and add soy sauce and wine mixture. Cook 3 to 4 minutes until sauce becomes thickened. Serve over hot rice.

Makes 4 servings.

Nutrient count per serving: 276 calories; 21 grams carbohydrate; 23 grams protein; 11 grams fat

Tuna Salad Niçoise

1 3-ounce can tuna
½ cup cooked French-style green
    beans (cold)
1 small potato, boiled and sliced
Lettuce
2 tablespoons Italian salad dressing

Arrange tuna, beans, and potato on a bed of lettuce. Drizzle with salad dressing.

Makes 1 serving.

Nutrient count per serving:
394 calories; 19 grams
carbohydrate; 19 grams fat

Oven "Fried" Fish

4 cups Corn Chex cereal
3 egg whites
½ cup skim milk
1 pound ocean perch fillets or other
    white fish

Preheat oven to 400°F. Blend cereal in a blender until fine. Transfer to a mixing bowl, and set aside.

In a small bowl, beat egg whites and skim milk until well blended. Dip fish fillets into egg mixture, then roll in cereal mixture, coating both sides.

Spray a cookie sheet several times with nonstick cooking spray. Spread fillets on cookie sheet. Lightly coat fillets with cooking spray. Bake 20 minutes or until fish flakes easily with a fork.

Makes 4 servings.

Nutrient count per serving:
219 calories; 23 grams
carbohydrate; 26 grams protein;
3 grams fat

Quick Catfish Creole

1 pound catfish fillets
1 24-ounce jar mild chunky salsa

Preheat oven to 400°F. Place fish fillets in an ungreased baking dish. Pour salsa over fish. Bake uncovered 25 minutes or until fish flakes easily with a fork. Serve over hot rice.

Makes 4 servings.

Nutrient count per serving:
172 calories; 11 grams
carbohydrate; 20 grams protein;
4 grams fat

Exercise Substitutions

If certain machine or cable exercises indicated for your shape-training routine aren't available at your workout facility, you may need to substitute exercises. Or you may want to vary your routine by trying a different exercise every so often. The following charts list exercises that can be interchanged with each other. For example, suppose your routine calls for machine chin-ups, but your gym doesn't have this equipment. Refer to the chart for back exercises, and you'll see that you can substitute negative chin-ups (under Free Weights/Generic) or wide-grip pulldowns (another machine exercise).

Thigh Exercises

Free Weights/Generic	Machine/Cable	Nonapparatus
Regular barbell squat	Leg press	Freehand squat
Dumbbell squat	Leg extension	Lunge to the front or side without weight
Wide-stance barbell squat	Close-stance leg press	
Close-stance half squat	Close-stance hack squat	
Dumbbell lunge to the front	Medium-stance hack squat	
Dumbbell lunge to the side		
Dead lift		

Buttocks Exercises

Free Weights/Generic	Machine/Cable	Nonapparatus
Dumbbell bun burner	Hip/hamstring curl	Do-anywhere bun burner
Reverse hyperextension		

Hamstring Exercises

Free Weights/Generic	Machine/Cable	Nonapparatus
Incline back kick on slant board	Leg curl	Assisted leg curl
	Pulley leg curl	
	Single-leg curl	
	Standing leg curl	

Back Exercises

Free Weights/Generic	Machine/Cable	Nonapparatus
Bent-over barbell row	Low seated row	
Dumbbell rowing	High-pulley row	
Negative chin-up	Machine chin-up	
Dumbbell pullover	Wide-grip pulldown	
	Close-grip front pulldown	

Chest Exercises

Free Weights/Generic	Machine/Cable	Nonapparatus
Dumbbell bench press	Machine bench press	Chair push-up
Barbell bench press	Cable crossover	
Decline bench press	Machine chest fly	
Incline dumbbell press		
Incline dumbbell fly		
Chest circles		
Floor dumbbell fly		

Shoulder Exercises

Free Weights/Generic	Machine/Cable	Nonapparatus
Dumbbell overhead press	Machine shoulder press	Lateral raise with books or with a partner
One-arm-at-a-time dumbbell overhead press	Machine lateral raise	
Barbell shoulder press		
Seated alternating dumbbell press		
Lateral raise		
Incline lateral raise		
Bench lateral raise		
Side lateral raise		
Incline side lateral raise		
Rear lateral raise		
Front lateral raise		
Upright row		

Biceps

Free Weights/Generic	Machine/Cable	Nonapparatus
Barbell curl	Machine curl	Biceps curl with books or with a partner
Concentration curl	Cable biceps curl	
Inner-biceps curl		
Seated alternating dumbbell curl		
Lying dumbbell curl		

Triceps Exercises

Free Weights/Generic	Machine/Cable	Nonapparatus
Close-grip bench press	Triceps pressdown	Chair dip
Bench dip	Machine dip	
Overhead triceps extension	Low-pulley triceps extension	
Dumbbell triceps kickback	Single-arm pulley pressdown	

Abdominal Exercises

Free Weights/Generic	Machine/Cable	Nonapparatus
Dumbbell side bend	Twisting leg raise on a dip stand	Twisting crunch
Side crunch	Knee-up on a dip stand	Broomstick crunch
Seated reverse crunch	Abdominal crunch machine	Floor crunch
Abdominal crunch with weight	Pulley crunch	Crunch up a wall
Decline bench crunch		

Calf Exercises

Free Weights/Generic	Machine/Cable	Nonapparatus
Calf raise on stairs or steps, using dumbbells	Seated calf raise	Calf raise on stairs or steps
	Standing calf raise	

References

Chapter 1: A Shortcut to Shape

"Calories Aren't Created Equal." *Mayo Clinic Health Letter,* March 1992, p. 7.

Hallum, R. "Body Double with the Golden Girls." *MuscleMag International,* May/June 1991, pp. 24–27, 121.

Hilgus, L. "Lipid in the Gut." *Men's Fitness,* August 1994, pp. 74–75, 110–112.

"Spot Reduction." *Muscle & Fitness,* February 1987, p. 10.

Uhlenbrock, D. "From Chubby to Champion." *Performance Press,* July 1994, pp. 12–13, 20.

Wang, N., R. S. Hikida, R. S. Staron, and J. A. Simoneau. "Muscle Fiber Types of Women After Resistance Training: Quantitative Ultrastructure and Enzyme Activity." *Pfluegers Archives of the European Journal of Physiology,* 424(5–6) (September 1993), pp. 494–502.

Chapter 2: Size Up Your Size

Jensen, M. D. "Research Techniques for Body Composition Assessment." *Journal of the American Dietetic Association,* 92(4) (April 1992), pp. 454–459.

Orphanidou, C., L. McCargar, C. L. Birmingham, J. Mathieson, and E. Goldner. "Accuracy of Subcutaneous Fat Measurement: Comparison of Skinfolds, Ultrasound, and Computed Tomography." *Journal of the American Dietetic Association,* 94(8) (August 1994), pp. 855–858.

Chapter 3: Your Health and the Shape of Fat

"Adiposity, Fat Distribution and Cardiovascular Risk." *American Family Physician,* 41(3) (March 1990), pp. 962–963.

Edwards, D. D. "Body Shape: In the Eye of the Receptor?" *Science News,* 133 (January 23, 1988), pp. 54–55.

"Even Love Handles Unhealthy, Says New Study." *Evansville Courier,* September 14, 1995, p. 1.

"Few Extra Pounds Called No Big Deal." *Evansville Courier,* September 15, 1995, p. 12.

Folsom, A. R., S. A. Kaye, T. A. Sellers, et al. "Body Fat Distribution and Five-Year Risk of Death in Older Women." *Journal of the American Medical Association,* 269(4) (January 27, 1993), pp. 483–487.

Petrek, J. A., M. Peters, C. Cirrincione, D. Rhodes, and D. Bajorunas. "Is Body Fat Topography a Risk Factor for Breast Cancer?" *Annals of Internal Medicine,* 118(5) (March 1, 1993), pp. 356–362.

Potera, C. "Exercise and Breast Cancer." *The Physician and Sportsmedicine,* 23(1) (January 1995), pp. 37–38.

Seim, H. C., and K. B. Holtmeier. "Effects of a Six-Week, Low-Fat Diet on Serum Cholesterol, Body Weight, and Body Measurements." *Family Practice Research Journal,* 12(4) (December 1992), pp. 411–419.

Shapira, D. V., N. B. Kumar, and G. H. Lyman. "Variation in Body Fat Distribution and Breast Cancer Risk in the Families of Patients with Breast Cancer and Control Families." *Cancer,* 71(9) (May 1993), pp. 2,764–2,768.

Stamford, B. "Apples and Pears." *The Physician and Sportsmedicine,* 19(1) (January 1991), pp. 123–124.

Swanson, C. A., N. Potischman, G. D. Wilbanks, L. B. Twiggs, et al. "Relation of Endometrial Cancer Risk to Past and Contemporary Body Size and Body Fat Distribution." *Cancer Epidemiology,* 2(4) (July–August 1993), pp. 321–327.

"Upper-Body Fat Distribution and Endometrial Cancer Risk." *Cancer Weekly,* October 14, 1991, pp. 26–27.

Chapter 4: Shape-Training Basics

Nichols, J. F., D. K. Omizo, K. K. Peterson, and K. P. Nelson. "Efficacy of Heavy-Resistance Training for Active Women over Sixty: Muscular Strength, Body Composition, and Program Adherence." *Journal of the American Geriatrics Society,* 41(3) (March 1993), pp. 205–210.

Whatley, J. E., W. J. Gillespie, J. Honig, M. J. Walsh, et al. "Does the Amount of Endurance Exercise in Combination with Weight Training and a Very-Low-Energy Diet Affect Resting Metabolic Rate and Body Composition?" *American Journal of Clinical Nutrition*, 59(5) (May 1994), pp. 1,088–1,092.

Chapter 5: Shape-Training Aerobics

"An After-Dinner Walk Speeds Weight Loss." *Prevention*, April 1984, p. 96.

Gall, S. L. "Swim Fins—Adding Splash to the Laps." *The Physician and Sportsmedicine*, 18(11) (November 1990), pp. 91–96.

"How to Burn 50 Percent More Calories." *1001 Weight Loss Secrets*, Fall 1995. p. 4.

Koszuta, L. E. "Can Fitness Be Found at the Top of the Stairs?" *The Physician and Sportsmedicine*, 15(2) (February 1987), pp. 165–169.

Koszuta, L. E. "Low-Impact Aerobics: Better than Traditional Aerobic Dance?" *The Physician and Sportsmedicine*, 14(7) (July 1986), pp. 156–161.

Miller, J. F., and B. A. Stamford. "Intensity and Energy Cost of Weight Walking vs. Running for Men and Women. *Journal of Applied Physiology*, 62(4) (April 1987), pp. 1,497–1,501.

Chapter 7: The H-Frame: Whittling Away Your Waist

Kohrt, W. M., K. A. Obert, and J. O. Holloszy. "Exercise Training Improves Fat Distribution Patterns in 60- to 70-Year-Old Men and Women." *Journal of Gerontology*, 47(4) (July 1992), pp. 99–105.

Rodin, J., N. Radke-Sharpe, M. Rebuffe-Scrive, and M. R. Greenwood. "Weight Cycling and Fat Distribution." *International Journal of Obesity*, 14(4) (April 1990), pp. 303–310.

Zarrow, S., and L. Rao. "Shrink Your Belly Bulge." *Prevention*, May 1992, pp. 33–35, 105–107.

Chapter 8: The I-Frame: Adding Curves in All the Right Places

Clark, N. "Athletes with Amenorrhea." *The Physician and Sportsmedicine*, 21(4) (April 1993), pp. 45–48.

Hakkinen, K., and M. Kallinene. "Distribution of Training Volume into One or Two Daily Sessions and Neuromuscular Adaptations in Female Athletes." *Electromyography and Clinical Neurophysiology*, 34(2) (March 1994), pp. 117–124.

Michielli, D. W., C. C. Dunbar, and M. I. Kalinski. "Is Exercise Indicated for the Patient Diagnosed as Anoretic?" *Journal of Psychosocial Nursing and Mental Health Services*, 32(8) (August 1994), pp. 33–35.

Thornton, J. S. "How Can You Tell When an Athlete Is Too Thin?" *The Physician and Sportsmedicine,* 18(12) (December 1990), pp. 124–133.

Chapter 9: The O-Frame: Paring Off Pounds

Gwinup, G. "Effect of Exercise Alone on the Weight of Obese Women." *Archives of Internal Medicine,* 135(5) (May 1975), pp. 676–680.

Gwinup, G. "Weight Loss Without Dietary Restriction: Efficacy of Different Forms of Aerobic Exercise." *American Journal of Sports Medicine,* 15(3) (May/June 1987), pp. 275–279.

Schelkin, P. H. "Treating Overweight Patients." *The Physician and Sportsmedicine,* 21(2) (February 1993), pp. 148–153.

Work, J. A. "Exercise for the Overweight Patient." *The Physician and Sportsmedicine,* 18(7) (July 1990), pp. 113–122.

Chapter 13: Shape-Training Nutrition

Zarrow, S., and L. Rao. "Shrink Your Belly Bulge." *Prevention,* May 1992, pp. 33–35, 105–107.

Appendix A: Shape Training During Pregnancy

White, J. "Exercising for Two: What's Safe for the Active Pregnant Woman?" *The Physician and Sportsmedicine,* 20(5) (May 1992), pp. 179–186.

About the Authors

Robert Kennedy, a leading authority on exercise and fitness, is the author of more than 30 top-selling books on these subjects, including *Pumping Up, Built! The New Bodybuilding for Everyone*, and *Reps*. In addition, he is the publisher of his own magazine, *MuscleMag International*.

Maggie Greenwood-Robinson is one of the country's best-known fitness authors. She has coauthored many books on fitness and nutrition, including *Lean Bodies, 50 Workout Secrets, High Performance Nutrition* and *Built! The New Bodybuilding for Everyone* (with Robert Kennedy). She writes frequently for many national fitness magazines.